Dosage
Calculation
Practice
for Nurses

Dosage Calculation Practice for Nurses

BONITA E. BROYLES, RN, BSN, EdD

THOMSON

DELMAR LEARNING

Australia Canada Mexico Singapore Spain United Kingdom United States

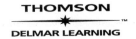

THOMSON

DELMAR LEARNING

Dosage Calculation Practice for Nurses

Bonita E. Broyles

Health Care Publishing Director:
William Brottmiller

Acquisitions Editor:
Matthew Kane

Executive Marketing Manager:
Dawn F. Gerrain

Executive Editor:
Cathy L. Esperti

Editorial Assistant:
Shelley Esposito

Production Editor:
James Zayicek

NOTICE TO THE READER

Contents

Preface

INTRODUCTION

A vital part of the nurse's role in providing safe medication administration to clients is the assurance that the client receives the accurate dose of each medication. Frequently this task involves dosage calculations. The nurse needs to ensure that the dose ordered by the health care provider is accurately calculated using the dosage form available and the dosage ordered. The instruction of nurses, in this crucial function, is an integral part of nursing education. The nurse must practice solving dosage calculations to become proficient at this skill.

To accurately perform dosage calculations, the nurse must understand

- basic mathematical calculations of addition, subtraction, multiplication, and division,
- common conversions used in dosage calculations
- Roman numerals that are used in medication orders
- how to calculate dosages of a variety of medication forms and routes

Dosage Calculation Practice for Nurses is a unique text containing over 1000 dosage calculation problems designed to provide ample practice in the mathematical calculations necessary for safe nursing practice. This text can be used in conjunction with any dosage calculation text or as a stand-alone practice text. It can also function as a resource test bank for faculty to develop dosage calculation quizzes and exams. Each unit contains 100 or more questions specific to the calculation topic of the unit. References at the end of the text are noted to ensure accuracy of drugs, dosages, and dosage forms used in the practice problems.

ORGANIZATION OF TEXT

The text begins with a table of standard conversion equivalents used when performing dosage calculations. Nine units of representative dosage problems follow this. Unit X is a comprehensive exam as a final review that includes the types of problems from the first nine units. The units contain problems covering the following areas:

Unit I: Mathematics Reviews
     a. Roman numerals, percents to decimals, fractions to percents
     b. Conversions

Unit II   Oral Dosage Calculations—Tablets and Capsules

Unit III   Oral Dosage Calculations—Liquid Preparations

Unit IV   Parenteral Medications—Subcutaneous, Intramuscular, and IV Bolus

Unit V   Calculating Dosages Using Powder or Crystalline-Form Drugs Requiring Reconstitution

Unit VI   Intravenous Infusion—Calculating Infusion Rates

Unit VII Intravenous Infusions—Calculating Flow Rates Using Drip Factors

Unit VIII Calculating Pediatric Dosages Using Body Weight and Body Surface Area

Unit IX   Advanced Calculations

Unit X   Comprehensive Exam

Each unit contains 100 or more dosage calculations specific to that content area, and the answers to the calculations for each are located at the end of that unit. The answers to the problems do not include the "work" associated with arriving at the proper conclusion. This is in the interest of eliminating any perception of bias of one calculation method over another. Each problem contains commonly ordered drugs and presents dosage forms and dosages congruent with those ordered by health care providers. Abbreviations used are also consistent with current practice. References used to ensure currency of drugs, dosage forms, and dosages are located at the end of the text.

About the Author

Dr. Broyles began her nursing career in 1968, working as a student nursing assistant while pursuing her Bachelor of Science degree in nursing from Ohio State University in Columbus, Ohio. She graduated with her BSN in 1970 and spent the next thirteen years staffing and teaching in obstetrics and gynecology. From 1972–1976, she taught in the Associate Degree Nursing Education program at Columbus Technical Institute (which is now Columbus State). During her 5-year position as Patient Teaching and Discharge Planning Coordinator for Obstetrics at Mt. Carmel Medical Center in Columbus (1976–1981), she published her first professional writing. At this juncture, she decided to expand both her mind and nursing skills into the medical-surgical arena of nursing where she has staffed and taught nursing since 1981. With her husband, Roger, she moved to North Carolina in 1985. She has been teaching in the nursing education department of Piedmont Community College in Roxboro, North Carolina since 1986 and is currently the course coordinator for Maternal-Child Nursing (teaching the pediatric nursing component of the course), Adult Nursing II, and Pharmacology. She is involved in both levels of nursing education in the Associate Degree Nursing Program with special emphasis on second-level nursing courses. She received her Master of Arts in Educational Media from North Carolina Central University in 1988, and her Doctorate of Education from LaSalle University in 1996. Her dissertation research concerned critical thinking in Associate Degree Nursing Students and was the largest study published on this topic. Dr. Broyles has since published nursing texts in the areas of pediatrics and pharmacology, and co-authored a pediatric test bank.

Acknowledgements

The author wishes to express her appreciation to all who contributed to the development of this text. Without the love, support, and encouragement of my husband, Roger, this project would not have come to completion.

The author also wishes to thank Matt Kane from Delmar Learning for his vision of this project and for affording the author the wonderful opportunity to do this work. His support during the writing of this text is greatly appreciated.

The Piedmont Community College Associate Degree Nursing students have consistently served as inspiration for the author's writings, making each a work of the heart.

The author wishes to thank the reviewers for their wonderful comments and suggestions. Having been a book reviewer for six years, Dr. Broyles appreciates the time and effort of the reviewers as they shared their expertise to help make this text user friendly and complete.

REVIEWERS

Susan Harrell, RN, MSN
Associate Professor
Doña Ana Branch Community College
Las Cruces, NM

Betty Kehl Richardson, RN, PhD, CS
Professor, Vocational Nursing Program
Austin Community College
Austin, Texas

David Leach
Professor, Mathematics
Jefferson College
Hillsboro, MO

Beverly Meyers
Professor, Mathematics
Jefferson College
Hillsboro, MO

Conversion Table

The following conversions are used in this text. Although pharmacology books may vary slightly in their conversions, these are the conversion values used by this author.

1. 1 liter (L) = 1000 milliliters (ml)

2. 1 ounce (oz) = 30 milliliters (ml)

3. 1 teaspoon (tsp) = 5 milliliters (ml)

4. 1 tablespoon (tbs) = 15 milliliters (ml)

5. 1 gram (g) = 1000 milligrams (mg)

6. 1 milligram (mg) = 1000 micrograms (mcg)

7. 1 grain (gr) = 60 milligrams (mg)

8. 1 kilogram (kg) = 2.2 pounds (lb)

9. 1/150 grain (gr) = 0.4 milligrams (mg)

10. 1/200 grain (gr) = 0.3 milligrams (mg)

Mathematics Review

ROMAN NUMERALS, PERCENTS, & FRACTIONS

1a. Roman numerals—Convert Arabic numbers to Roman numerals.

1. 3	= _____			14. 19	= _____
2. 5	= _____			15. 6	= _____
3. 10	= _____			16. 2	= _____
4. 14	= _____			17. 8	= _____
5. 20	= _____			18. 29	= _____
6. 9	= _____			19. 40	= _____
7. 100	= _____			20. 51	= _____
8. 7	= _____			21. 35	= _____
9. 500	= _____			22. 39	= _____
10. 1000	= _____			23. 59	= _____
11. 4	= _____			24. 70	= _____
12. 90	= _____			25. 15	= _____
13. 32	= _____				

PERCENTS—CONVERT PERCENTS TO DECIMALS.

1. 10% = _____
2. 25% = _____
3. 50% = _____
4. 15% = _____
5. 22% = _____
6. 75% = _____
7. 5% = _____
8. 2½ % = _____
9. 1% = _____
10. 37½ % = _____
11. 7% = _____
12. 11% = _____
13. 67% = _____

14. 2% = _____
15. 13% = _____
16. 98% = _____
17. 6% = _____
18. 42% = _____
19. 36% = _____
20. 12½ % = _____
21. 53% = _____
22. 85% = _____
23. 24% = _____
24. 90% = _____
25. 71% = _____

FRACTIONS—CONVERT FRACTIONS TO PERCENTS.

1. ¼ = _____
2. ½ = _____
3. ¾ = _____
4. 1 ½ = _____
5. 1/50 = _____
6. 1/400 = _____
7. 1/8 = _____
8. 12 ½ = _____

9. 1/25 = _____
10. 2 ½ = _____
11. 25 ½ = _____
12. 2/3 = _____
13. 1/10 = _____
14. 9/10 = _____
15. 7/8 = _____
16. 1/5 = _____

17. 3/10   = _____

18. 2/5   = _____

19. 1/200   = _____

20. 1/150   = _____

21. 15½   = _____

22. 3/5   = _____

23. 1/20   = _____

24. 7/10   = _____

25. 4/5   = _____

CONVERSIONS

1b. Convert the following problems.

1. ¼ gr   = _____ mg

2. 30 ml   = _____ oz

3. 0.06 gm   = _____ gr

4. 300 mcg   = _____ mg

5. 1 ½ oz   = _____ ml

6. 5 cc   = _____ ml

7. 10 ml   = _____ tsp

8. 1500 ml   = _____ L

9. 4 L   = _____ ml

10. 1½ gr   = _____ mg

11. 0.050 mg   = _____ mcg

12. 1000 ml   = _____ pt

13. 250 mcg   = _____ mg

14. 2 tsp   = _____ ml

15. 30 kg   = _____ lb

16. 12 oz   = _____ ml

17. 165 lb   = _____ kg

18. 3 gr   = _____ mg

19. 0.5 g   = _____ mg

20. 120 mg   = _____ g

21. 1.25 L   = _____ ml

22. 55 lb   = _____ kg

23. 45 ml   = _____ oz

24. 2.5 g   = _____ mg

25. 3 tsp   = _____ ml

26. 1/150 gr   = _____ mg

27. 0.3 mg   = _____ gr

28. 1000 mg   = _____ g

29. 6 oz   = _____ ml

30. ½ gr   = _____ mg

31. 1 g   = _____ mg

32. 44 lb   = _____ kg

33. 78 kg   = _____ lb

34. 1 mg   = _____ mcg

35. 60 ml   = _____ oz

36. 2 L   = _____ ml

37. 40 kg   = _____ lb

38. 60 mg   = _____ gr

39. 1 C   = _____ oz

40. 1 qt   = _____ oz

41. 1/6 gr   = _____ mg

42. 500 ml   = _____ pt

43. 1 tsp   = _____ ml

44. 15 ml   = _____ tsp

45. 2 tsp   = _____ ml

46. 200 mg   = _____ g

47. 0.01 mg   = _____ mcg

48. 21 oz   = _____ ml

49. 90 kg   = _____ lb

50. 0.09 g   = _____ gr

51. 2 pt   = _____ oz

52. 2 tbsp   = _____ tsp

53. 224 lb   = _____ kg

54. 1 ½ tsp   = _____ ml

55. 3000 ml   = _____ L

56. 0.125 mg   = _____ mcg

57. 75 mcg   = _____ mg

58. 16 oz   = _____ pt

59. 2 qt   = _____ oz

60. 60 in   = _____ cm

Answers for Unit I

1a. Roman Numerals

1. III or iii	
2. V or v	
3. X or x	
4. XIV or xiv	
5. XX or xx	
6. IX or ix	
7. C or c	
8. vii or VII	
9. D or d	
10. M or m	
11. IV or iv	
12. XC or xc	
13. XXXII or xxxii	
14. XIX or xix	
15. VI or vi	
16. II or ii	
17. VIII or viii	
18. XXIX or xxix	
19. XL or xl	
20. LI or li	
21. XXXV or xxxv	
22. XXXIX or xxxix	
23. LIX or lix	
24. LXX or lxx	
25. XV or xv	

Percents

1. 0.1
2. 0.25
3. 0.5
4. 0.15
5. 0.22
6. 0.75
7. 0.05
8. 0.025
9. 0.01
10. 0.375
11. 0.07
12. 0.11
13. 0.67
14. 0.02
15. 0.13
16. 0.98
17. 0.06
18. 0.42
19. 0.36
20. 0.125
21. 0.53
22. 0.85
23. 0.24
24. 0.9
25. 0.71

Fractions

1. 25%
2. 50%
3. 75%
4. 150%
5. 2%
6. 0.25%
7. 12.5%
8. 1250%
9. 4%
10. 250%
11. 2550%
12. 66.7% or 66 2/3%

13. 10%
14. 90%
15. 87.5%
16. 20%
17. 30%
18. 40%
19. 0.5%
20. 0.7%
21. 1550%
22. 60%
23. 5%
24. 70%
25. 80%

1b. Conversions

1. 15 mg
2. 1 oz
3. 1 gr
4. 0.3 mg
5. 45 ml
6. 5 ml
7. 2 tsp
8. 1.5 L
9. 4000 ml
10. 90 mg
11. 50 mcg
12. 2 pt
13. 0.25 mg
14. 10 ml

15. 66 lb
16. 360 ml
17. 75 kg
18. 180 mg
19. 500 mg
20. 0.12 g
21. 1250 ml
22. 25 kg
23. 1.5 oz
24. 2500 mg
25. 15 ml
26. 0.4 mg
27. 1/200 gr
28. 1 g

29. 180 ml
30. 30 mg
31. 1000 mg
32. 20 kg
33. 171.6 lb
34. 1000 mcg
35. 2 oz
36. 2000 ml
37. 88 lb
38. 1 gr
39. 8 oz
40. 32 oz
41. 10 mg
42. 1 pt
43. 5 ml
44. 3 tsp

45. 10 ml
46. 0.2 g
47. 10 mcg
48. 630 ml
49. 198 lb
50. 1½ gr
51. 32 oz
52. 6 tsp
53. 101.8 kg
54. 7.5 ml
55. 3 L
56. 125 mcg
57. 0.075 mg
58. 1 pt
59. 64 oz
60. 150 cm

Oral Dosage Calculations— Tablets and Capsules

Fill in the correct answers to the following problems.

1. The physician writes an order for secobarbital 0.2 g prn for sleep. Each secobarbital capsule is labeled 100 mg. The nurse should administer _____ capsule(s) per dose.

2. The physician prescribes phenytoin 100 mg po each day. On hand are phenytoin capsules labeled 0.1 gram. The nurse should administer _____ capsule(s) per dose.

3. The physician prescribes acyclovir 0.8 g po q4h. On hand are acyclovir tablets labeled 200 mg. The nurse should administer _____ tablet(s) for each dose.

4. The physician prescribes alprazolam 1 mg po tid. On hand are 0.5 mg alprazolam tablets. The nurse should administer _____ tablet(s) per dose.

5. The physician prescribes 600 mg of acyclovir po q4h. On hand are acyclovir tablets labeled 200 mg. The nurse should administer _____ tablet(s) per day.

6. The physician orders 0.2 mg of misoprostol. On hand are 200 mg misoprostol tablets. The nurse should administer _____ tablet(s) per dose.

7. The physician orders pemoline 37.5 mg po qAM. The pharmacy sends 18.75 premoline tablets. The nurse should administer _____ tablet(s) per dose.

8. The physician orders diltiazem hydrochloride SR gr 1½ po bid. On hand are diltiazem HCl SR labeled capsules labeled 90 mg per capsule. The nurse should administer _____ capsule(s) per dose.

9. The physician orders phenobarbital gr 1⅔ po q12h. On hand are 100 mg phenobarbital tablets. The nurse should administer _____ tablet(s) per dose.

20. The physician orders verapamil hydrochloride 120 mg po q6h. On hand are 2 gr vera-pamil tablets. The nurse should administer _____ tablet(s) per dose.

21. The physician orders celecoxib 200 mg po in 2 divided doses per day. On hand are 100 mg celecoxib capsules. The nurse should administer _____ capsule(s) per dose.

22. The physician orders fexofenadine 120 mg po in 2 divided doses per day. Available are 60 mg fexofenadine capsules. The nurse should administer _____ capsule(s) per dose.

23. The physician orders auranolin 3 mg q8h po. On hand are 6 mg scored tablets of aura-nolin. The nurse should administer _____ tablet(s) per dose.

24. The physician orders ibuprofen 800 mg po every 6 hours for pain. On hand are 400 mg ibuprophen caplets. The nurse should administer _____ caplet(s) per dose.

25. The physician orders digoxin 0.25 mg po qAM. On hand are 125 mcg digoxin tablets. The nurse should administer _____ tablet(s) every morning after counting the client's apical pulse.

26. The physician orders diflunisal 0.5 g po q12h. Available are 250 mg diflunisal tablets. The nurse should administer _____ tablet(s) per dose.

27. The physician orders 0.15 mg of levothroid to be administered by mouth each morning. The pharmacy sends 150 mcg levothroid tablets. The nurse should administer _____ tablet(s) for each dose.

28. The physician orders 500 mg of amoxicillin by mouth to be administered every 6 hours. Available are 250 mg amoxicillin capsules. The nurse should administer _____ capsule(s) for each dose. The nurse will administer how many capsules per day? _____ .

29. The physician orders carbidopa/levodopa 20/200 tid. On hand are 10/100 carbidopa/levodopa tablets. The nurse should administer _____ tablet(s) per day.

30. The physician orders carisoprodol 1400 mg per day in 4 divided doses. On hand are 350 mg carisoprodol tablets. The nurse should administer _____ tablet(s) per dose.

31. The physician orders digoxin .125 mg once a day. The pharmacy sends 125 mcg digoxin tablets. The nurse should administer _____ tablet(s) once a day.

32. The physician orders carvedilol 3.125 mg bid. The pharmacy sends the nurse 6.25 mg carvedilol tablets. The nurse should administer _____ tablet(s) per dose.

33. The physician orders oxycodone 5 mg/acetaminophen (APAP) 325 mg combined tablets, one every 4 hours as needed for pain. The pharmacy has on hand 5 mg/APAP 325 mg oxycodone tablets. The nurse can administer a maximum of _____ tablets in a 24 hour period.

34. The physician orders cefaclor .5 g every 8 hours. The pharmacy sends 250 mg cefaclor capsules. The nurse should administer _____ capsule(s) per dose.

35. The physician orders cefadroxil monohydrate 1 g/day in a single dose. The pharmacy sends 500 mg cefadroxil monohydrate capsules. The nurse should administer _____ capsule(s) per dose.

36. The physician orders cefpodoxime proxetil 400 mg a day in two divided doses. The nurse should administer _____ mg per dose.

37. The physician orders celecoxib 200 mg in two divided doses per day. The pharmacy sends 100 mg celecoxib capsules. The nurse should administer _____ capsule(s) per dose.

38. The physician orders cerivastatin 400 mcg once a day. The pharmacy sends 0.2 mg cerivastatin tablets. The nurse should administer _____ tablet(s) per day.

39. The physician orders cetirizine hydrochloride 10 mg once a day. The pharmacy sends tablets 5 mg cetirizine hydrochloride. The nurse should administer _____ tablet(s) per day.

40. The physician orders chlorambucil 0.1–0.2 mg/kg in a single daily dose. The client weighs 140 pounds. What is the maximum daily dose this client can receive? _____ .

41. The physician orders chlordiazepoxide 25 mg tid by mouth. The pharmacy sends 5 mg chlordiazepoxide capsules. The nurse should administer _____ capsule(s) per dose.

42. The physician orders hydrochlorothiazide 12.5 mg by mouth each day. The pharmacy sends 25 mg hydrochlorothiazide tablets. The nurse should administer _____ tablet(s) per day.

43. The physician orders chlorothiazide 1.5 g bid. The pharmacy sends 500 mg chlorothiazide tablets. The nurse should administer _____ tablet(s) per dose.

44. The physician orders chlorpheniramine maleate 24 mg in 4 divided doses per day. The pharmacy sends 4 mg chlorpheniramine maleate tablets. The nurse should administer _____ tablet(s) per dose.

45. The physician orders bexarotene 300 mg per day as a single oral dose. The pharmacy sends 75 mg bexarotene tablets. The nurse should administer _____ tablet(s) per daily dose.

46. The physician orders dofetilide 0.250 mg bid. The pharmacy sends 125 mcg dofetilide capsules. The nurse should administer _____ capsule(s) per dose.

47. The physician orders oxcarbazepine 600 mg bid. The pharmacy fills the prescription with 150 mg oxcarbazepine tablets. When placing tablets in the client's daily pill container, the home health nurse counts out _____ tablets per day.

48. The physician orders zolpidem tartrate 10 mg every day at bedtime. The pharmacy sends 10 mg zolpidem tartrate tablets. The nurse should administer _____ tablet(s) per dose.

49. The physician orders zolmitriptan 1250 mcg by mouth tid. The pharmacy sends 2.5 mg zolmitriptan tablets. The nurse should administer _____ tablet(s) per dose.

50. The physician orders zidovudine 0.1 g every 4 hours. The pharmacy fills the prescription with 100 mg zidovudine capsules. The home health nurse should instruct the client to take _____ capsule(s) every 4 hours totaling _____ capsule(s) per day.

51. The physician orders lorazepam 1 mg every 6 hours as needed for anxiety. The pharmacy places 0.5 mg lorazepam tablets in the controlled substances. The nurse should administer _____ tablet(s) per dose.

52. The physician orders codeine sulfate 30 mg every 4 hours by mouth as needed for pain. The pharmacy stocks ½ gr codeine sulfate tablets in the controlled substances. The nurse should administer _____ tablet(s) for each dose requested.

53. The physician orders 0.01 g of zaleplon by mouth at bedtime. The pharmacy sends 10 mg zaleplon capsule(s). The nurse should administer _____ capsule(s) per dose.

54. The physician orders oxycontin ⅓ gr every 12 hours by mouth for 7 days. The pharmacy stocks the controlled substances with 20 mg oxycontin tablets. The nurse should administer _____ tablet(s) per dose.

55. The physician orders zalcitabine 0.75 mg by mouth tid. What is the total daily dose of zalcitabine ordered? _____

56. The physician orders zafirlukast 0.020 g by mouth bid. The pharmacy sends 10 mg zafirlukast tablets. The nurse should administer _____ tablet(s) per dose.

57. The physician orders MS contin ¼ gr tablets by mouth every 4 hours for chronic pain. The pharmacy stocks the controlled substances with 15 mg MS contin tablets. The nurse should administer _____ tablet(s) per dose.

58. The physician orders codeine sulfate 1 gr every 6 hours by mouth as needed for pain. The pharmacy stocks the controlled substances with 30 mg codeine sulfate tablets. The nurse should administer _____ tablet(s) per dose.

59. The physician orders clindamycin 5 gr every 6 hours by mouth. On hand are 300 mg clinidamycin tablets. The nurse should administer _____ tablet(s) per dose.

60. The physician orders clofibrate 500 mg by mouth qid. The pharmacy sends 0.5 g clofibrate capsules. The nurse should administer _____ capsule(s) per dose.

61. The physician orders clonazepam 0.25 mg by mouth qAM. The pharmacy fills the client's prescription with 125 mcg clonazepam tablets. The nurse should instruct the client to take _____ tablet(s) every _____ .

62. The physician orders clonidine 100 mcg bid by mouth. The pharmacy fills the client's prescription with 0.1 mg clonidine tablets. The nurse should instruct the client to take _____ tablet(s) per day.

63. The physician orders amoxicillin 0.5 g qid by mouth for 10 days. The pharmacy fills the client's prescription with 500 mg amoxicillin capsules. The nurse should instruct the client to take _____ capsule(s) per dose.

64. The physician orders amoxicillin 0.5 g qid by mouth for 10 days. The pharmacy fills the client's prescription with 500 mg amoxicillin capsules. The client should take _____ capsule(s) to complete the entire prescription.

65. The physician orders morphine sulfate 60 mg slow release tablets by mouth daily. The pharmacy fills the client's prescription with ½ gr tablets of slow release morphine sulfate. The nurse should instruct the client to take _____ tablet(s) per dose.

66. The physician orders warfarin sodium 5 mg by mouth every day. The pharmacy sends 2.5 mg warfarin sodium tablets. The nurse should administer _____ tablet(s) per dose.

67. The physician orders verapamil 4 gr qd by mouth. The pharmacy fills the client's prescription with 240 mg verapamil tablets. The nurse should instruct the client to take _____ tablet(s) per day.

68. The physician orders veniafaxine hydrochloride 75 mg/day in 3 divided doses. The client should receive _____ mg per dose.

69. The physician orders vancomycin hydrochloride 2 g/day by mouth in 4 divided doses. The pharmacy fills the client's prescription with 500 mg vancomycin hydrochloride capsules. The nurse should instruct the client to take _____ capsule(s) per dose.

70. The physician orders vancomycin hydrochloride 0.5 g/day by mouth in four divided doses. The pharmacy fills the client's prescription with 125 mg vancomycin hydrochloride capsules. The nurse should instruct the client to take _____ capsule(s) per dose.

71. The physician orders valsartan 320 mg by mouth daily. Available are 160 mg valsartan capsules. The nurse should administer _____ capsule(s) per dose.

72. The physician orders acetaminophen 325 mg every 4 hours by mouth as needed for pain. The pharmacy supplies 325 mg acetaminophen tablets. The nurse should instruct the client to take _____ tablet(s) every 4 hours as needed for pain.

73. The physician orders valproic acid 250 mg tid po. The pharmacy fills the prescription with 250 mg valproic acid tablets. The nurse should instruct the client to take _____ tablet(s) per dose.

74. The physician orders valacyclovir hydrochloride 1 g po tid for 7 days. The pharmacy fills the client's prescription with 500 mg valacyclovir hydrochloride tablets. The nurse should instruct the client to take _____ tablet(s) per dose.

75. The physician orders ursodiol 1 g po in 2 divided doses per day. The client weighs 220 pounds and the safe dosage range is 8–10 mg/kg/day. The pharmacy fills the client's prescription with 500 mg ursodiol tablets. Is the ordered dose safe for this client? _____ Yes _____ No

76. The physician orders ursodiol 0.9 g po in 3 divided doses per day. The pharmacy fills the client's prescription with 300 mg ursodiol capsules. The nurse should instruct the client to take _____ capsule(s) per dose.

77. The physician orders trovafloxacin mesylate 100 mg po qd for 7–10 days. The pharmacy sends 100 mg trovafloxacin mesylate tablets. The nurse should administer _____ tablet(s) per dose.

78. The physician orders trimethoprim 160 mg/sulfamethoxazole 800 mg po q12h. The pharmacy sends 80 mg trimethoprim/400mg sulfamethoxazole tablets. The nurse should administer _____ tablet(s) per dose.

79. The physician orders triazolam 125 mcg po before bedtime. The pharmacy sends 0.125 mg triazolam tablets. The nurse should administer _____ tablet(s) before bedtime.

80. The physician orders triamcinolone hexacetonide .004 g po tid. The pharmacy send 2 mg triamcinolone hexacetonide tablets. The nurse should administer _____ tablet(s) per dose.

81. The physician orders trazodone hydrochloride 75 mg po at hs. The pharmacy fills the client's prescription with 50 mg trazodone hydrochloride tablets. The nurse should instruct the client to take _____ tablet(s) per dose.

82. The physician orders pancrease 5 capsules po ac. The client should take the 5 capsules when? _____

83. The physician orders tamoxifen 0.02 g po bid. The pharmacy fills the client's prescription with 20 mg tamoxifen tablets. The nurse should instruct the client to take _____ tablet(s) twice a day.

84. The physician orders sulindac 0.3 g po in 2 divided doses. The pharmacy sends 150 mg sulindac tablets. The nurse should administer _____ tablet(s) per dose.

85. The physician orders clorazepate dipotassium 7.5 mg bid po. The pharmacy sends 3.75 mg clorazepate dipotassium tablets. The nurse should administer _____ tablet(s) per dose.

86. The physician orders clozapine 300 mg po daily. The pharmacy sends 5 gr clozapine tablets. The nurse should administer _____ tablet(s) per dose.

87. The physician orders colestipol hydrochloride 2000 mg bid po. The pharmacy fills the client's prescription with 1 g colestipol hydrochloride tablets. The nurse should instruct the client to take _____ tablet(s) per dose.

88. The physician orders cyclobenzaprine hydrochloride 40 mg/day po in 4 divided doses. The pharmacy fills the client's prescription with 10 mg cyclobenzaprine hydrochloride tablets. The nurse should instruct the client to take _____ tablet(s) per dose.

89. The physician orders diazepam 2.5 mg po bid. The pharmacy stocks the controlled substances with 5 mg diazepam tablets. The nurse should administer _____ tablet(s) per dose.

90. The physician orders doxycycline 100 mg po q12h. The pharmacy sends 0.1 g doxycycline capsules. The nurse should administer _____ capsule(s) per day.

91. The physician orders dolasetron mesylate 0.1g po 1 hour before chemotherapy. The pharmacy sends 50 mg dolasetron mesylate tablets. The nurse should administer _____ tablet(s) per dose.

92. The physician orders erythromycin 1 g day po in 3 divided doses. The pharmacy sends 333 mg erythromycin tablets. The nurse should administer _____ tablet(s) per dose.

93. The physician orders pyrodoxine 0.2 g po qd for rifampin-induced B6 deficiency. The pharmacy supplies 50 mg pyrodoxine tablets. The nurse should instruct the client to take _____ tablet(s) per dose.

94. The physician orders ferrous gluconate 0.325 g po qd. The pharmacy supplies 325 mg ferrous gluconate tablets. The nurse should administer _____ tablet(s) per dose.

95. The physician orders indomethacin 200 mg po qd. The pharmacy supplies 50 mg in-domethacin capsules. The client should be instructed to take _____ capsule(s) per day.

96. The physician orders lithium carbonate 1.2 g po qd in 4 divided doses. The pharmacy supplies 300 mg lithium carbonate capsules. The nurse should instruct the client to take _____ tablet(s) per dose.

97. The physician orders lorazepam 2 mg po bid prn for anxiety. The pharmacy supplies 0.5 mg lorazepam tablets. The client should be instructed to take _____ tablet(s) per dose.

98. The physician orders naproxen sodium .75 g po qd. The pharmacy supplies 375 mg naproxen sodium tablets. The nurse should instruct the client to take _____ tablet(s) per dose.

99. The physician orders nitroglycerin sublingual 600 mcg at first sign of a heart attack. The pharmacy supplies the client with sublingual 0.3 mg nitroglycerin tablets. The client should place _____ tablet(s) under his or her tongue at the first sign of a heart at-tack.

100. The physician orders propylthiouracil 300 mg po qd in 4 divided doses. The pharmacy supplies 50 mg propylthiouracil tablets. The nurse should instruct the client to take _____ tablet(s) per dose.

101. The physician orders phenobarbital 1½ gr po qd. The pharmacy supplies 60 mg phenobarbital tablets in the controlled substances. The nurse should instruct the client to take _____ tablet(s) per dose.

Answers for Unit II

1. 2 capsules
2. 1 capsule
3. 4 tablets
4. 2 tablets
5. 18 tablets/day
6. 1 tablet
7. 2 tablets
8. 1 capsule
9. 1 tablet
10. 2 capsules
11. 1 tablet
12. 2 tablets
13. 2 tablets
14. 1 tablet
15. 1 capsule
16. 1 tablet
17. 2 tablets
18. 1 tablet
19. 2 tablets
20. 1 tablet
21. 1 capsule
22. 1 capsule
23. ½ tablet
24. 2 caplets
25. 2 tablets
26. 2 tablets
27. 1 tablet
28. 2 capsules/dose; 8 capsules/day
29. 6 tablets/day
30. 1 tablet
31. 1 tablet
32. ½ tablet
33. 6 tablets
34. 2 capsules
35. 2 capsules
36. 200 mg
37. 1 capsule
38. 2 tablets
39. 2 tablets
40. 12.7 mg
41. 5 capsules
42. ½ tablet
43. 3 tablets
44. 1½ tablets
45. 4 tablets
46. 2 capsules
47. 8 tablets/day
48. 1 tablet
49. ½ tablet
50. 1 capsule every 4 hours totaling 6 capsules/day
51. 2 tablets
52. 1 tablet
53. 1 capsule

54. 1 tablet
55. 2.25 mg
56. 2 tablets
57. 1 tablet
58. 2 tablets
59. 1 tablet
60. 1 capsule
61. 2 tablets every morning
62. 2 tablets
63. 1 capsule
64. 40 capsules
65. 2 tablets
66. 2 tablets
67. 1 tablet
68. 25 mg
69. 1 capsule
70. 1 capsule
71. 2 capsules
72. 1 tablet
73. 1 tablet
74. 2 tablets
75. Yes
76. 1 capsule
77. 1 tablet
78. 2 tablets
79. 1 tablet
80. 2 tablets
81. 1½ tablets
82. before meals
83. 1 tablet
84. 2 tablets
85. 2 tablets
86. 1 tablet
87. 2 tablets
88. 1 tablet
89. ½ tablet
90. 2 capsules
91. 2 tablets
92. 1 tablet
93. 4 tablets
94. 1 tablet
95. 4 capsules
96. 1 tablet
97. 4 tablets
98. 2 tablets
99. 2 tablets
100. 1½ tablets
101. 1½ tablets

Oral Dosage Calculations—Liquid Preparations

NOTE: When rounding decimals in dosage calculations, round the **final answer** to the nearest tenth.

1. The physician writes an order for acetaminophen 240 mg po for an elderly adult. You have on hand 80 mg acetaminophen oral liquid in 0.8 ml. The nurse should administer _____ ml per dose.

2. The physician orders acetaminophen 280 mg po for a child. You have on hand acetaminophen 80 mg per 2.5 ml in oral liquid. The nurse should administer _____ ml per dose.

3. The physician orders 180 mg acyclovir po. The pharmacy supplies acyclovir suspension 200 mg/5 ml. The nurse should administer _____ ml per dose.

4. The physician orders amoxicillin 275 mg po. The pharmacy supplies amoxicillin suspension 250 mg/5ml. The nurse should administer _____ ml per dose.

5. The physician orders amoxicillin 350 mg po. The pharmacy filled the prescription with amoxicillin suspension 400 mg/5 ml. The nurse should instruct the client to take_____ ml. per dose.

6. The physician orders amphetamine sulphate 20 mg tid for attention deficit disorder. The pharmacy supplies 10 mg tablets. The client is unable to swallow tablets so the nurse crushes each tablet in 2 ml of water and a drop of cherry syrup. The nurse should administer _____ ml for each dose.

7. The physician orders 1200 mg amprenavir bid po. The pharmacy supplies amprenavir oral liquid 15 mg/ml for this client who is unable to swallow capsules. The nurse should administer _____ ml per dose.

8. The physician orders atovaquone 1.5 g po once daily. The pharmacy fills the client's prescription with atovaquone 750 mg/5 ml suspension. The client should be instructed to take_____ ml per dose.

9. The physician orders amoxicillin/potassium clavulanate 100 mg po q12h. The pharmacy fills the client's prescription with amoxicillin/potassium clavulanate 125 mg/5 ml suspension. The client's parent should be instructed to administer _____ ml per dose.

10. The physician orders azithromycin 300 mg qd for 5 days po. The pharmacy fills the client's prescription with azithromycin 200 mg/5ml. The nurse should instruct the client's parent to administer _____ ml per daily dose.

11. The physician orders acetaminophen 320 mg po for a child's temperature elevation. The mother purchases acetaminophen liquid 80 mg/2.5 ml. The mother should administer _____ tsp per dose.

12. The physician orders amoxicillin 250 mg po. The pharmacy supplies amoxicillin suspension 250 mg/5ml. The nurse should instruct the client to take _____ tsp per dose.

13. The physician orders 1350 mg amprenavir bid po. The pharmacy supplies amprenavir oral liquid 15 mg/ml. The nurse should instruct the client to take _____ oz per dose.

14. The physician orders cefaclor 2 g via gastric tube in 2 divided doses. The pharmacy sends cefaclor 375 mg/5 ml suspension. The nurse should administer _____ ml per dose.

15. The physician orders cefadroxil monohydrate 750 mg po bid for a child weighing 50 kg. The pharmacy sends cefadroxil monohydrate 500 mg/5 ml. The nurse should administer _____ ml per dose.

16. The physician orders cefpodoxime proxetil 200 mg q12h po. The pharmacy sends cefpodoxime proxetil 100 mg/5 ml. The nurse should administer _____ ml/dose and _____ ml per day.

17. The physician orders ceprozil 112.5 mg po bid for 10 days for a child weighing 15 kg. The pharmacy sends ceprozil suspension 125 mg/5 ml. The nurse should administer _____ ml per dose.

18. The physician orders cefaclor 750 mg po qd for 10 days for a child weighing 25 kg. The pharmacy fills the prescription with cefaclor 187 mg/5 ml suspension. The mother should be instructed to administer _____ ml per daily dose.

19. The physician orders digoxin elixir 125 mcg po each day. The pharmacy sends digoxin 0.05 mg/ml. The nurse should administer _____ ml per dose after monitoring the client's apical pulse.

20. The physician orders ceftibuten 400 mg po qd. The pharmacy sends ceftibuten suspension 190 mg/5ml. The nurse should administer _____ ml per daily dose.

21. The physician orders cephalexin hydrochloride 4 g in 4 divided doses po each day for 5 days. The pharmacy supplies cephalexin hydrochloride suspension 250 mg/5 ml. The nurse should instruct the client to take _____ ml per dose.

22. The physician orders digoxin 0.25 mg po qd. The pharmacy sends digoxin elixer 0.05 mg/ml. The nurse should administer _____ ml per dose.

23. The physician orders cephradine 500 mg q6h po for 7 days. The pharmacy fills the prescription with cephradine suspension 250 mg/ml per the client's request. The client should be instructed to take _____ ml per dose.

24. The physician orders chlorothiazide suspension 0.3 g po each day. The pharmacy fills the prescription with chlorothiazide suspension 250 mg/5 ml. The daily dose for this client is _____ ml.

25. The physician orders 200 mg acetaminophen po every 4 hours for a young child. The parent purchases acetaminophen suspension containing 80 mg/0.8 ml. The child's dose is _____ ml.

26. The physician orders clarithromycin suspension 275 mg po bid. The pharmacy sends clarithromycin suspension 250 mg/5 ml. The client should receive _____ ml per dose.

27. The physician orders clemastine fumarate po 8 mg qd. The pharmacy supplies clemastine fumarate syrup 0.5 mg/5 ml. The client should be instructed to take _____ ml per daily dose.

28. The physician orders clindamycin HCl 300 mg po q6h. The pharmacy supplies clindamycin HCl 75 mg/ 5 ml oral solution. The client should be instructed to take _____ ml per dose.

29. The physician orders clonazepam 5 mg tid po for a client with severe Parkinson's disease. The pharmacy supplies 2 mg tablets. Because the client cannot swallow tablets, the nurse crushes each tablet in 3 ml of water making a concentration of 2 mg/3 ml. The client should receive _____ ml per dose of this solution to receive the ordered dose.

30. The physician orders cloxacillin sodium 110 mg q6h po. The pharmacy fills the prescription with cloxacillin sodium oral solution 125 mg/5 ml. The client should receive _____ ml per dose.

31. The physician orders codeine sulfate ½ gr po. The pharmacy supplies the controlled substances with codeine sulfate oral solution 15 mg/5 ml. The nurse should administer _____ ml per dose.

32. The physician orders diazepam 2 mg po. In the controlled substances, diazepam is stocked in tablets as well as oral solution. The oral solution is 5 mg/ml. The nurse decides to use the oral solution and administers _____ ml per dose.

33. The physician orders digoxin elixir 0.125 mg po qAM. The digoxin elixir is 0.05 mg/ml. The nurse should administer _____ ml per dose.

34. The physician orders docusate sodium 100 mg per gastric tube bid. The docusate sodium liquid is 150 mg/15 ml. The nurse should administer _____ ml per dose per gastric tube.

35. The physician orders doxepin HCl 150 mg po qhs. The pharmacy fills the prescription with doxepin HCl liquid 10 mg/ml. The client should be instructed to take _____ ml at what time? _____

36. The physician orders doxycycline monohydrate 200 mg/day in 2 divided doses po. The pharmacy fills the prescription with doxycycline monohydrate oral syrup 50 mg/5 ml. The client should be instructed to take _____ ml per dose.

37. The physician orders erythromycin 125 mg po qid. The pharmacy fills the prescription with erythromycin suspension 200 mg/5 ml. The client should be instructed to take _____ ml every six hours.

38. The physician orders phenytoin 150 mg po bid. The pharmacy sends phenytoin suspension 100 mg/4 ml. The nurse should administer _____ ml per dose.

39. The physician orders docusate sodium 10 mg po bid. The pharmacy supplies docusate sodium syrup 150 mg/15 ml. The nurse should administer _____ ml per dose.

40. The physician orders diazepam 1 mg solution po. The oral solution is 5 mg/ml. The nurse should administer _____ ml per dose.

41. The physician orders 75 mcg of digoxin elixir po qd. The pharmacy supplies digoxin elixir 0.05 mg/ml. The nurse should administer _____ ml per dose.

42. The physician orders docusate sodium 100 mg po bid. The pharmacy sends docusate sodium 200 mg/5ml. The nurse should administer _____ ml per dose.

43. The physician orders doxycycline monohydrate syrup 60 mg po in 3 divided doses per day. The pharmacy fills the prescription with doxycycline monohydrate syrup 50 mg/5 ml. The client should be instructed to take _____ ml per dose. In order to achieve the ordered daily dose the client should receive _____ ml in 3 divided doses per day.

44. The physician orders erythromycin 300 mg po tid. The pharmacy sends erythromycin suspension 250 mg/5 ml. The nurse should administer _____ ml per dose.

45. The physician orders phenytoin 300 mg po bid. The pharmacy fills the prescription with phenytoin suspension per the client's request with a concentration of 125 mg/5 ml. The client should be instructed to take _____ ml per dose twice a day.

46. The physician orders famotidine 20 mg po bid. The pharmacy supplies famotidine suspension with a concentration of 40 mg/5 ml. The nurse should administer _____ ml per dose.

47. The physician orders felbamate 600 mg po tid. The pharmacy fills the prescription with felbamate suspension 400 mg/5 ml. The client should be instructed to take _____ ml per dose.

48. The physician orders ferrous gluconate oral solution 300 mg per gastric tube bid. The pharmacy supplies ferrous gluconate 150 mg/2.5 ml. The nurse should administer _____ ml per gastric tube bid.

49. The physician orders ferrous sulfate 115 mg po qd. Ferrous sulfate is supplied in tablet as well as syrup form. The client elects to buy the ferrous sulfate syrup 90 mg/5ml. The client should be instructed to take _____ ml per day.

50. The physician orders fluconazole 150 mg po. The pharmacy supplies fluconazole suspension 200 mg/5ml. The nurse should administer _____ ml per dose.

51. The physician orders fluoxetine HCl 45 mg po qd. The pharmacy fills the client's prescription with fluoxetine HCl oral solution (per client's request) 20 mg/5 ml. The client should be instructed to take _____ ml per day.

52. The physician orders furosemide 40 mg po bid. Because the client has a gastric tube and is receiving nothing by mouth, the nurse contacts the physician and has the ordered route changed to "per gastric tube." The pharmacy sends furosemide oral solution 10 mg/ml. The nurse should administer _____ ml per dose.

53. The physician orders phenobarbital 200 mg po per day in 2 divided doses. The controlled substances has phenobarbital elixir 20 mg/5 ml. The nurse should administer _____ ml per dose.

54. The physician orders griseofulvin 0.5 g po qd in 2 divided doses. The pharmacy fills the prescription with griseofulvin oral suspension 125 mg/5 ml. The client should be instructed to take _____ ml per dose.

55. The physician orders guaifenesin syrup 100 mg q4h for cough. The guaifenesin syrup is supplied in a concentration of 50 mg/5ml. The client should take _____ tsp per dose.

56. The physician orders haloperidol 3 mg po at hs. The pharmacy fills the prescription with haloperidol oral concentrate 2 mg/ml. The client should be instructed to take _____ ml at bedtime.

57. The physician orders hydrochlorothiazide 20 mg po qd. The pharmacy fills the prescription with hydrochlorothiazide oral solution 50 mg/5 ml. The client should be instructed to take _____ ml per day.

58. The physician orders oxycodone elixir 5 mg q4h for pain. The oxycodone elixir is supplied in a concentration of 5 mg/5 ml. The client should receive _____ ml per dose.

59. The physician orders hydromorphone HCl 10 mg po q4h for severe pain. Hydromorphone oral liquid is supplied as 1 mg/ml. The client should be instructed to take _____ ml per dose.

60. The physician orders felbamate 300 mg po qid. The pharmacy supplies felbamate suspension 600 mg/5 ml. The nurse should administer _____ ml per dose.

61. The physician orders fluconazole 135 mg po qd. The pharmacy fills the prescription with fluconazole oral suspension 50 mg/5ml. The client's parent should be instructed to administer _____ ml per day.

62. The physician orders furosemide 100 mg po now. The pharmacy sends furosemide oral solution 40 mg/5 ml. The nurse should administer _____ ml now.

63. The physician orders hydrochlorothiazide 25 mg po qd. The pharmacy sends hydrochlorothiazide oral solution 50 mg/5 ml. The nurse should administer _____ ml per daily dose.

64. The physician orders guaifenesin oral liquid 300 mg q4h. The guaifenesin oral liquid is supplied in a concentration of 200 mg/5 ml. The client should be instructed to take _____ ml every 4 hours.

65. The physician orders oxycodone 10 mg q4h po prn pain. The oxycodone elixir is supplied in a concentration of 5 mg/5 ml. The client should be instructed to take _____ tsp per dose.

66. The physician orders phenobarbital elixir 60 mg po bid. The pharmacy fills the prescription with phenobarbital elixir 20 mg/5 ml. The client's parent should be instructed to administer _____ ml per dose.

67. The physician orders griseofulvin oral suspension 0.75 g once a day po. The pharmacy fills the prescription with griseofulvin suspension 125 mg/5 ml. The client should receive _____ ml per day.

68. The physician orders guaifenesin syrup 150 mg po q4h for cough. The guaifenesin syrup is supplied in a concentration 50 mg/5 ml. The client should be instructed to take _____ ml or _____ tsp per dose.

69. The physician orders haloperidol 0.5 mg oral solution po bid. The pharmacy fills the prescription with haloperidol oral solution 2 mg/ 2 ml. The client should be instructed to take _____ ml per dose.

70. The physician orders hydromorphone 2.5 mg po q4h for pain. The pharmacy supplies the controlled substances with hydromorphone oral liquid 1 mg/ml. The nurse should administer _____ ml per dose.

71. The physician orders hydroxyzine HCl 50 mg po qid. The pharmacy sends hydroxyzine HCl syrup 10 mg/5 ml. The nurse should administer _____ ml per dose.

72. The physician orders ibuprofen 400 mg po tid. The pharmacy sends ibuprofen suspension 100 mg/5 ml. The client should receive _____ ml per dose.

73. The physician orders indomethacin sodium 50 mg po bid. The pharmacy fills the prescription with indomethacin sodium suspension 25 mg/4 ml. The client should be instructed to take _____ ml per dose.

74. The physician orders hydroxyzine HCl 40 mg po qd in 4 divided doses. The pharmacy fills the prescription with hydroxyzine HCl syrup 10 mg/5 ml. The client's parent should be instructed to administer _____ tsp per dose.

75. The physician orders ibuprofen 150 mg po q4h for fever > 38 C. The pharmacy supplies ibuprofen oral suspension 50 mg/1.25 ml. The client should receive _____ ml per dose.

76. The physician orders isoniazid 300 mg po qd. The pharmacy fills the prescription with isoniazid syrup (per client request) 50 mg/5 ml. The client should be instructed to take _____ oz per dose.

77. The physician orders isoniazid 300 mg po qd. The pharmacy supplies isoniazid syrup 50 mg/5 ml. The nurse should administer _____ ml per daily dose.

78. The physician orders itraconazole oral solution 200 mg po qd. The pharmacy has in stock itraconazole 10 mg/ml oral solution. The client should take _____ ml per daily dose.

79. The physician orders lamivudine oral solution 150 mg po bid. The pharmacy sends lamivudine 5 mg/ml to the nursing unit. The nurse should administer _____ ml per dose.

80. The physician orders meperidine HCl 75 mg po q4h as needed for pain. The pharmacy fills the prescription meperidine HCl 50 mg/5 ml syrup (per client request). The client should be instructed to take _____ tsp per dose.

81. The physician orders metaproterenol sulfate 20 mg po qid. The pharmacy sends metaproterenol sulfate syrup 10 mg/5 ml. The client should receive _____ ml per day.

82. The physician orders methadone HCl 2.5 mg q3–4h po as needed for pain. The pharmacy supplies the controlled substances with methadone HCl 5 mg/5 ml. The client should receive _____ ml per dose.

83. The physician orders theophylline elixir 225 mg po q8h. The pharmacy fills the prescription with theophylline elixir 150 mg/15 ml. The client should be instructed to take _____ ml per dose.

84. The physician orders zidovudine syrup 100 mg q4h po. The pharmacy fills the prescription with zidovudine syrup 10 mg/ml. The client should be instructed to take _____ ml per dose.

85. The physician orders vancomycin HCl 0.125 g po q6h. The pharmacy supplies vancomycin HCl 250 mg/5 ml oral solution. The nurse should administer _____ ml per dose.

86. The physician orders valproic acid syrup 900 mg po tid. The pharmacy supplies valproic acid syrup 250 mg/5 ml. The client should receive _____ ml per dose.

87. The physician orders tramadol HCl 75 mg po q4h prn for pain. The pharmacy supplies tramadol HCL 25 mg/5 ml. The client should be instructed to take _____ tsp per dose.

88. The physician orders theophylline oral solution 75 mg qid po. The pharmacy supplies theophylline 80 mg/15 ml oral solution. The client should be instructed to take _____ ml per dose.

89. The physician orders tetracycline HCl 500 mg po qid. The pharmacy fills the prescription with tetracycline HCl syrup (per client request) 125 mg/5 ml. The client should be instructed to take _____ ml per dose.

90. The physician orders temazepam 30 mg oral solution po at hs for an elderly client. The pharmacy fills the prescription with temazepam 7.5 mg/ml oral solution. The client should be instructed to take _____ ml at bedtime.

91. The physician orders sulfisoxazole suspension 3 g po loading dose then 2 g po q6h. The pharmacy supplies sulfisoxazole suspension 500 mg/5 ml. The client should be instructed to take _____ oz loading dose and then _____ ml per dose every 6 hours.

92. The physician orders sucralfate suspension 1 g po qid. The pharmacy supplies sucralfate suspension 500 mg/5 ml. The client should take _____ ml per dose.

93. The physician orders stavudine oral solution 30 mg po bid. The pharmacy supplies powder for oral solution to be reconstituted to concentration of 1 mg/ml. The client should receive _____ ml per dose.

94. The physician orders sodium polystyrene sulfonate 10 g po bid to client in renal failure. The pharmacy supplies sodium polystyrene sulfonate 15g/60 ml suspension. The client should receive _____ ml per dose.

95. The physician orders sirolimus 15 mg po loading dose followed by 5 mg/day maintenance dose. The pharmacy supplies sirolimus in oral solution 1 mg/ml. The client should
receive _____ ml loading dose followed by _____ ml daily maintenance
dose.

96. The physician orders sacrosidase 17,000 IU po qd. The pharmacy supplies sacrodidase
8500 IU/ml. The client should receive _____ ml per daily dose.

97. The physician orders ritonavir oral solution 1.2 g po qd in 2 divided doses. The pharmacy
supplies ritonavir oral solution 600 mg/7.5 ml. The client should receive _____ ml
per dose.

98. The physician orders prednisone oral solution 20 mg po qid. The pharmacy supplies
prednisone oral solution 5 mg/5 ml. The client should receive _____ ml per dose.

99. The physician orders morphine syrup 30 mg po q4h for pain. The pharmacy fills the
client's prescription with morphine syrup 20 mg/ml. The hospice nurse should instruct
the client's family to administer _____ ml per dose for pain.

100. The physician orders minocycline HCl 200 mg po initial dose followed by 100 mg q12h. The pharmacy fills the prescription with minocycline HCl syrup 50 mg/5 ml. The client should be instructed to take _____ ml for initial dose followed by _____ ml every 12 hours.

Answers for Unit III

1.	2.4 ml	28.	20 ml
2.	8.8 ml	29.	7.5 ml
3.	4.5 ml	30.	4.4 ml
4.	5.5 ml	31.	10 ml
5.	4.4 ml	32.	0.4 ml
6.	4 ml	33.	2.5 ml
7.	80 ml	34.	10 ml
8.	10 ml	35.	15 ml; at bedtime
9.	4 ml	36.	10 ml
10.	7.5 ml	37.	3.125 or 3.1 ml
11.	2 tsp	38.	6 ml
12.	1 tsp	39.	1 ml
13.	3 oz	40.	0.2 ml
14.	13.3 ml	41.	1.5 ml
15.	7.5 ml	42.	2.5 ml
16.	10 ml and 20 ml	43.	2 ml; 6 ml
17.	4.5 ml	44.	6 ml
18.	20.1 ml	45.	12 ml
19.	2.5 ml	46.	2.5 ml
20.	10.5 ml	47.	7.5 ml
21.	20 ml	48.	5 ml
22.	5 ml	49.	6.4 ml
23.	2 ml	50.	3.8 ml
24.	6 ml	51.	11.3 ml
25.	2 ml	52.	4 ml
26.	5.5 ml	53.	25 ml
27.	80 ml	54.	10 ml

55. 2 tsp
56. 1.5 ml
57. 2 ml
58. 5 ml
59. 10 ml
60. 2.5 ml
61. 13.5 ml
62. 12.5 ml
63. 2.5 ml
64. 7.5 ml
65. 2 tsp
66. 15 ml
67. 30 ml
68. 15 ml; 3 teaspoons
69. 0.5 ml
70. 2.5 ml
71. 25 ml
72. 20 ml
73. 8 ml
74. 1 tsp
75. 3.8 ml
76. 1 oz
77. 30 ml
78. 20 ml
79. 30 ml
80. 1½ tsp
81. 10 ml
82. 2.5 ml
83. 22.5 ml
84. 10 ml
85. 2.5 ml
86. 18 ml
87. 3 tsp
88. 14.1 ml
89. 20 ml
90. 4 ml
91. 1 oz; 20 ml
92. 10 ml
93. 30 ml
94. 40 ml
95. 15 ml; 5 ml
96. 2 ml
97. 7.5 ml
98. 20 ml
99. 1.5 ml
100. 20 ml; 10 ml

Parenteral Medications—Subcutaneous, Intramuscular, and IV Bolus

Fill in the correct answers for the following problems.

1. The physician orders 10 units of regular insulin and 15 units of NPH insulin SC qAM. What is the total number of units of insulin the nurse will draw up in the syringe and administer? _____

2. The physician orders 14 units of regular insulin and 28 units of NPH insulin SC at 1700 hours. What is the total number of units of insulin the nurse will draw up in the syringe and administer? _____

3. The physician orders 40 units of 70/30 insulin to be administered SQ qAM. The nurse must use a standard syringe because no insulin syringe is available. The label on the 70/30 insulin says there are 100 u/ml. The nurse will administer _____ ml SC.

4. The physician orders atropine 1/150 gr SC. The atropine vial is labeled 0.4 mg/ml. The nurse should administer _____ ml SC.

5. The physician orders scopolamine 0.3 mg SC. The scopolamine vial is labeled 1/200 gr/ml. The nurse should administer _____ ml SC.

6. The physician orders amikacin sulfate 300 mg IM. The amikacin sulfate IM solution comes in a concentration of 250 mg/ml. The nurse will administer _____ ml of amikacin sulfate.

7. The physician orders morphine sulfate 2 mg IV now. The morphine sulfate tubex contains 4 mg/ml. The nurse should administer _____ ml IV bolus.

8. The physician orders amitriptyline HCl 30 mg IM stat. The amitriptyline injectable comes in a concentration of 10 mg/ml. The nurse should administer _____ ml.

9. The physician orders 450 IU of antihemophilic factor (Factor VIII) IV qd. The pharmacy supplies the antihemophilic factor in a concentration of 75 IU/5 ml. The nurse should administer _____ ml IV bolus.

10. The physician orders kanamycin sulfate 0.4 g IM. The vial label on the kanamycin sulfate states 500 mg/2 ml. The nurse should administer _____ ml IM.

11. The physician orders ardeparin sodium 7500 U SC bid. The vial label on the ardeparin sodium reads 5000 u/0.5 ml. The nurse should administer _____ ml SC.

12. The physician orders amikacin sulfate 500 mg IM. The amikacin sulfate IM solution contains 250 mg/ml. The nurse should administer _____ ml IM.

13. The physician orders amikacin 125 mg IM. The amikacin sulfate IM solution comes in a concentration of 62.5 mg/ml. The nurse should administer _____ ml.

14. The physician orders naxolone HCl 0.002 g IV. The naloxone HCl comes in a 10 ml vial labeled 1mg/ml. The nurse should administer _____ ml IV.

15. The physician orders morphine sulfate 1.5 mg IV. The tubex containing the morphine sulfate contains 2 mg/ml. The nurse should administer _____ ml IV.

16. The physician orders 2500 U heparin sodium SC bid. The pharmacy sends heparin sodium 10,000 U/ml. The nurse should administer _____ ml SC.

17. The physician orders promethazine sulfate 25 mg IV. The label on the vial containing the promethazine sulfate states 25 mg/ml. The IV drug resource states that each 12.5 mg of promethazine sulfate should be diluted with 5 ml of normal saline for injection prior to administration. The nurse should administer a total fluid and medication bolus of _____ ml.

18. The physician orders ardeparin sodium 8000 U SC bid. The pharmacy supplies ardeparin sodium 10,000 U/0.5 ml. The nurse should administer _____ ml SC.

19. The physician orders heparin sodium 3000 U SC bid prophylaxis. The pharmacy supplies heparin sodium 5000 U/0.5 ml. The client should receive _____ ml SC bid.

20. The physician orders enoxaparin sodium 30 mg SC bid. The pharmacy sends enoxaparin sodium 60 mg/0.6 ml. The client should receive _____ ml SC bid.

21. The physician orders enoxaparin sodium 50 mg SC qd. The pharmacy sends enoxiparin sodium 100 mg/ml. The nurse should administer _____ ml SC each day.

22. The physician orders atropine sulfate 0.6 mg SC q6h. The pharmacy sends atropine sulfate 1/150 gr/0.5 ml. The client should receive _____ ml SC q6h.

23. The physician orders ketorolac tromethamine 30 mg IV q6h for 48 hours. The client should receive a total of how many doses of ketorolac tromethamine? _____

24. The physician orders enoxaparin sodium 40 mg SC qd. The pharmacy sends enoxaparin sodium 40 mg/0.4 ml. The client should receive _____ ml SC each day.

25. The physician orders ketorolac tromethamine 30 mg IV q6h for 48 hours. The pharmacy sends ketorolac tromethamine 15 mg/ml. The nurse should administer _____ ml as an IV bolus.

26. The physician orders heparin sodium 7000 U SC bid. The pharmacy sends heparin sodium 5000 U/0.5 ml. The nurse should administer _____ ml SC bid.

27. The physician orders 0.3 mg atropine sulfate SC q4h. The pharmacy sends atropine sulfate 0.6 mg/ml. The nurse should administer _____ ml SC q4h.

28. The physician orders 1/100 gr atropine sulfate q6h SC. The pharmacy sends atropine sulfate 0.6 mg/ml. The client should receive _____ ml SC q6h.

29. The physician orders ketorolac tromethamine 15 mg IV q6h for 48 hours post-operatively. The pharmacy supplies ketorolac tromethamine 30 mg/ ml. The nurse should administer _____ ml IV bolus.

30. The physician orders bethanechol chloride 5 mg tid SC. The pharmacy supplies bethanechol chloride 5 mg/ml. The client should receive _____ ml SC tid.

31. The physician orders bleomycin sulfate 2 units IV bolus. The pharmacy sends reconstituted bleomycin sulfate 15 U/5ml. The nurse should administer _____ ml IV bolus.

32. The physician orders ceftazidime 2 g IV bolus. The pharmacy sends reconstituted ceftazidime 1 g/10 ml. The nurse should administer _____ ml over 6–10 minutes IV bolus.

33. The physician orders cyanocobalamin 50 mcg IM. The pharmacy sends cyanocobalamin 100 mcg/ml. The client should receive _____ ml IM.

34. The physician orders desmopressin acetate 15 mcg SC in two divided doses. The pharmacy sends desmopressin acetate 15 mcg/ml. The nurse should administer _____ ml SC per dose.

35. The physician orders leucovorin calcium 25 mg IV bolus. The pharmacy sends leucovorin calcium 50 mg/5 ml. The nurse should administer _____ ml IV bolus.

36. The physician orders interferon alfa-2b recombinant 14 million U SC. The pharmacy sends interferon alfa-2b recombinant 10 million U/0.5 ml. The client should receive _____ ml SC.

37. The physician orders meperidine HCl 35 mg IM. The physician supplies the controlled substances with meperidine HCl 50 mg/ml. The client should receive _____ ml IM.

38. The physician orders bleomycin sulfate 45 U IV bolus. The pharmacy sends reconstituted bleomycin sulfate 30 U/10 ml. The nurse should administer _____ ml IV bolus.

39. The physician orders meperidine HCl 100 mg IM because the client has no intravenous access. The pharmacy supplies the controlled substances with meperidine HCL 75 mg/ml. The nurse should administer _____ ml IM.

40. The physician orders metoclopramide 10 mg IV bolus. The pharmacy supplies a meto-clopramide vial with 5 mg/ml. The nurse should administer _____ ml IV bolus over 2–3 minutes.

41. The physician orders ceftazidime 1 g IV bolus. The pharmacy sends reconstituted cef-tazidime 2g/20 ml. The nurse should administer _____ ml over 3–5 minutes IV bolus.

42. The physician orders meperidine HCl 40 mg IM. The pharmacy supplies the controlled substances with meperidine HCl 50 mg/ml. The nurse should administer _____ ml IM.

43. The physician orders cyanocobalamin 0.3 mg IM. The pharmacy sends cyanocobalamin 100 mcg/ 0.5 ml. The client should receive _____ ml IM.

44. The physician orders desmopressin acetate 8 mcg SC in 2 divided doses. The pharmacy sends desmopressin acetate 4 mcg/ml. The client should receive _____ ml SC per dose.

45. The physician orders 125 mg meperidine HCl IM because the client does not have an intravenous access. The pharmacy supplies the controlled substances with meperidine HCl 75 mg/ml. The nurse should administer _____ ml IM.

46. The physician orders dalteparin sodium 5000 U SC bid. The pharmacy supplies a vial labeled dalteparin sodium 10,000 U/ml. The nurse should administer _____ ml SC bid.

47. The physician orders metoclopramide 30 mg IV bolus as a premed for chemotherapy. The pharmacy supplies metoclopramide 5 mg/ml. The nurse should administer _____ ml slowly IV bolus.

48. The physician orders meperidine HCl 35 mg IM because the client does not have an IV access. The pharmacy supplies the controlled substances with meperidine HCl 25 mg/ml. The nurse should administer _____ ml IM.

49. The physician orders diazepam 5 mg IV bolus prior to cardioversion. The pharmacy supplies diazepam 5 mg/ml. The nurse should administer _____ ml very slowly IV bolus.

50. The physician orders dezocine 5 mg IV bolus q2–4 h for pain. The pharmacy supplies dezocine in the controlled substances as 10 mg/ml. The nurse should administer _____ ml as ordered.

51. The physician orders diazoxide IV 70 mg IV bolus. The pharmacy supplies diazoxide IV in a concentration of 15 mg/ml. The client should receive _____ ml as ordered.

52. The physician orders digoxin 50 mcg IV bolus. The pharmacy supplies digoxin 0.1 mg/ml. The client should receive _____ ml IV bolus.

53. The physician orders digoxin immune Fab 38 mg IV bolus. The pharmacy supplies digoxin immune Fab 10 mg/ml. The client should receive _____ ml IV bolus.

54. The physician orders droperidol 5 mg IM. The pharmacy sends droperidol 2.5 mg/ml. The client should receive _____ ml IM.

55. The physician orders lorazepam 1.5 mg IV bolus. The pharmacy supplies lorazepam 2 mg/ml. The nurse should administer _____ ml IV bolus.

56. The physician orders dexamethasone 10 mg IV bolus. The pharmacy supplies 4 mg/ml dexamethasone. The nurse should administer _____ ml IV bolus as ordered.

57. The physician orders estrogen conjugated parenteral 0.025 g IM. The pharmacy sends estrogen conjugated parenteral 25 mg/ml. The nurse should administer _____ ml IM.

58. The physician orders filgrastim 150 mcg SC. The pharmacy supplies filgrastim 300 mcg/ml. The client should receive _____ ml SC.

59. The physician orders furosemide 35 mg IV bolus. The pharmacy sends a 5 ml vial of furosemide 20 mg/ml. The nurse should administer _____ ml over 1½–2 minutes.

60. The physician orders dezocine 10 mg IV bolus q3h prn for pain. The pharmacy supplies controlled substances with dezocine 5 mg/ml. The client should receive _____ ml as ordered.

61. The physician orders diazepam 10 mg IV bolus prior to bronchoscopy. The pharmacy supplies diazepam 5 mg/ml. The client should receive _____ ml very slowly IV bolus.

62. The physician orders digoxin 125 mcg IV bolus. The pharmacy sends digoxin 0.25 mg/ml. The nurse should administer _____ ml IV bolus after monitoring apical pulse.

63. The physician orders .3 mg filgrastim SC. The pharmacy supplies filgrastim 300 mcg/ml. The nurse should administer _____ ml SC.

64. The physician orders furosemide 80 mg IV bolus over 4 minutes. The pharmacy supplies furosemide 20 mg/ml. The client should receive _____ ml IV bolus as ordered.

65. The physician orders dezocine 7.5 mg IV bolus q2h prn for pain. The pharmacy supplies the controlled substances with dezocine 15 mg/ml. The client should receive _____ ml as ordered.

66. The physician orders diazoxide IV 45 mg IV bolus. The pharmacy sends diazoxide IV in a concentration of 15 mg/ml. The client should receive _____ ml as ordered.

67. The physician orders digoxin 0.15 mg IV bolus. The pharmacy supplies digoxin 100 mcg/ml. The client should receive _____ ml IV bolus after monitoring apical pulse.

68. The physician orders lorazepam 2 mg IV bolus. The pharmacy supplies 0.001 g/ml of lorazepam. The nurse should administer _____ ml IV bolus as ordered.

69. The physician orders dexamethasone 6 mg IV bolus. The pharmacy supplies dexamethasone 4 mg/ml. The nurse should administer _____ ml IV bolus as ordered.

70. The physician orders furosemide 0.04 g IV bolus. The pharmacy sends furosemide 20 mg/ml. The client should receive _____ ml IV bolus.

71. The physician orders fluphenazine 15 mg SC. The pharmacy supplies fluphenazine 25 mg/ml. The nurse should administer _____ ml SC.

72. The physician orders folic acid 1000 mcg SC. The pharmacy sends folic acid 5 mg/ml. The client should receive _____ ml SC.

73. The physician orders 0.020 g glatiramer acetate SC qd. The pharmacy sends glatiramer acetate 20 mg/ml. The client should receive _____ ml SC.

74. The physician orders granisetron HCl 3 mg IV bolus. The pharmacy supplies granisetron HCl 1 mg/ml. The nurse should administer _____ ml IV bolus.

75. The physician orders histrelin acetate 350 mcg SC qd. The pharmacy supplies histrelin acetate 0.5 mg/ml. The client should receive _____ ml SC.

76. The physician orders hydralazine HCl 35 mg IV bolus. The pharmacy supplies hydralazine HCl 20 mg/ml. The nurse should administer _____ ml IV bolus.

77. The physician orders regular insulin 9 U and NPH insulin 34 U SC qAM. The nurse will administer a total of _____ U in a LO-DOSE® (U 50 u/½ ml) insulin syringe.

78. The physician orders lorazepam 1.5 mg IV bolus now. Lorazepam is supplied in a concentration of 4 mg/ml. The nurse should administer _____ ml IV bolus now.

79. The physician orders methylprednisolone 30 mg IV bolus q6h. The pharmacy sends methylprednisolone 20 mg/ml. The nurse should administer _____ ml q6h.

80. The physician orders lorazepam 0.004 g IV bolus. The pharmacy supplies lorazepam 2000 mcg/ml. The nurse should administer _____ ml IV bolus as ordered.

81. The physician orders naloxone HCl 0.4 mg IV bolus now. The pharmacy supplies naloxone HCl 0.02 mg/ml. The nurse should administer _____ ml IV bolus now.

82. The physician orders methylprednisolone 40 mg IV bolus q12h. The pharmacy sends methylprednisolone 0.08 g/2 ml. The nurse should administer _____ ml IV bolus q12h.

83. The physician orders promethazine HCl 12.5 mg IV bolus. The pharmacy supplies promethazine HCl 0.025 g/ml. According to your IV drug handbook, you should dilute the promethazine HCl with 10 ml of normal saline for each 25 mg of promethazine HCl to be administered. The nurse should administer a total of _____ ml of diluted solution to achieve the ordered dose.

84. The physician orders scopalamine hydrobromide 600 mcg IM on call to operating room (OCTOR). The pharmacy sends scopalamine hydrobromide 0.4 mg/ml. The client should receive _____ ml as ordered.

85. The physician orders somatropin 28 mg SC divided into 7 doses/week. The pharmacy supplies somatropin 5 mg/ml. The nurse should administer _____ ml SC per dose.

86. The physician orders spectinomycin HCl 2 g IM now. The clinic pharmacy supplies spectinomycin HCl 2g/5ml. The nurse should administer _____ ml divided into IM injections (and administered at the same time).

87. The physician orders sumatriptan succinate 6 mg SC now. The pharmacy supplies sumatriptan succinate 3 mg/0.25 ml. The nurse should administer _____ ml SC now.

88. The physician orders terbutaline sulfate 0.25 mg SC. The pharmacy sends terbutaline sulfate 1 mg/4ml. The nurse should administer _____ ml SC.

89. The physician orders tobramycin sulfate 80 mg IM q8h. The pharmacy supplies to-bramycin sulfate 0.04 g/ml. The nurse should administer _____ ml IM q8h.

90. The physician orders triamcinolone acetonide 5 mg IM qd. On hand is triamcinolone acetonide 3 mg/ml. The nurse should administer _____ ml IM qd.

91. The physician orders terbutaline sulfate 200 mcg SC. The pharmacy supplies terbutaline sulfate 1 mg/ml. The nurse should administer _____ ml SC.

92. The physician orders testosterone 40 mg IM 2–3 times weekly. Testosterone is supplied as 100 mg/ 2 ml. The nurse should administer _____ ml IM as ordered.

93. The physician orders triflupromazine HCl 60 mg IM now. The pharmacy supplies triflupromazine HCl 20 mg/ml. The nurse should administer _____ ml IM now.

94. The physician orders vasopressin 8 U subcutaneous bid. Vasopressin is supplied as 20 U/ml. The nurse should administer _____ ml SC bid.

95. The physician orders naloxone HCl 1.0 mg IV bolus now. The pharmacy sends naloxone HCl 0.4 mg/ml. The nurse should administer _____ ml IV bolus now.

96. The physician orders methylprednisolone 80 mg IV bolus now. The pharmacy sends methylprednisolone 20 mg/ml. The nurse should administer _____ ml IV bolus now.

97. The physician orders interferon alfa-2B recombinant 30 million U SC per week. Interferon alfa-2B recombinant is supplied as 10 million U/0.2 ml. The nurse should administer _____ ml SC as ordered.

98. The physician orders regular insulin 12 U and NPH insulin 28 U SC qAM. When drawing these insulins in the same syringe, which measures 100 U/ml, the nurse should administer _____ unit(s) SC as ordered.

99. The physician orders fentanyl citrate 0.1 mg IM on call to OR. The pharmacy supplies fentanyl citrate 0.05 mg/ml. The nurse should administer _____ ml IM as ordered.

100. The physician orders vasopressin 10 U SC tid. The pharmacy sends vasopressin 20 U/ml. The nurse should administer _____ ml SC tid.

Answers for Unit IV

1. 25 U
2. 42 U
3. 0.4 ml
4. 1 ml
5. 1 ml
6. 1.2 ml
7. 0.5 ml
8. 3 ml
9. 30 ml
10. 1.6 ml
11. 0.75 ml
12. 2 ml
13. 2 ml
14. 2 ml
15. 0.75 ml
16. 0.25 ml
17. 11 ml (1 ml of medication + 10 ml of normal saline)
18. 0.4 ml
19. 0.3 ml
20. 0.3 ml
21. 0.5 ml
22. 0.75 ml
23. 8 doses
24. 0.4 ml
25. 2 ml
26. 0.7 ml
27. 0.5 ml
28. 1 ml
29. 0.5 ml
30. 1 ml
31. 0.7 ml
32. 20 ml
33. 0.5 ml
34. 0.5 ml
35. 2.5 ml
36. 0.7 ml
37. 0.7 ml
38. 15 ml
39. 1.3 ml
40. 2 ml
41. 10 ml
42. 0.8 ml
43. 1.5 ml
44. 1 ml
45. 1.7 ml
46. 0.5 ml
47. 6 ml
48. 1.4 ml
49. 1 ml
50. 0.5 ml
51. 4.66 or 4.7 ml
52. 0.5 ml
53. 3.8 ml
54. 2 ml
55. 0.75 ml

56. 2.5 ml
57. 1 ml
58. 0.5 ml
59. 1.75 or 1.8 ml
60. 2 ml
61. 2 ml
62. 0.5 ml
63. 1 ml
64. 4 ml
65. 0.5 ml
66. 3 ml
67. 1.5 ml
68. 2 ml
69. 1.5 ml
70. 2 ml
71. 0.6 ml
72. 0.2 ml
73. 1 ml
74. 3 ml
75. 0.7 ml
76. 1.75 ml
77. 43 units
78. 0.375 or 0.38 ml

79. 1.5 ml
80. 2 ml
81. 2 ml
82. 1 ml
83. 5.5 ml (0.5 ml med + 5 ml normal saline)
84. 1.5 ml
85. 0.8 ml
86. 5 ml; 2 injections
87. 0.5 ml
88. 1 ml
89. 2 ml
90. 1.7 ml
91. 0.2 ml
92. 0.8 ml
93. 3 ml
94. 0.4 ml
95. 2.5 ml
96. 4 ml
97. 0.6 ml
98. a total of 40 units
99. 2 ml
100. 0.5 ml

Calculating Dosages Using Powder or Crystalline-Form Drugs Requiring Reconstitution

NOTE: When rounding decimals in dosage calculations, round off final answer to tenths, *EXCEPT* if answer is less than 1, then round off to hundredths. If answer is less than one milliliter, rounding to tenths may result in too much medication given.

1. The physician orders acyclovir 200 mg IV. A vial of 500 mg of acyclovir comes in powder form with directions to reconstitute with 5 ml of normal saline. How many milliliters would contain the ordered amount? _____

2. The doctor orders 112.5 mg of cefazolin IV. A 500 mg vial of cefazolin powder has instructions to reconstitute with 2 ml of sterile water. How many milliliters would contain the ordered amount? _____

3. The physician orders 500 mg of ceftazidime IV. The label on the 2 gram vial of ceftazidime reads to reconstitute with 10 ml of sterile water. How many milliliters would contain the ordered amount? _____

4. The label on the 1 g vial of ampicillin reads to reconstitute with sodium chloride to achieve a concentration of 125 mg/5 ml. How many milliliters of sodium chloride should be added to the vial to achieve this concentration? _____

5. The label on the 2 g vial of ampicillin reads to reconstitute with sodium chloride to achieve a concentration of 1000 mg/ 100 ml. How many milliliters of sodium chloride should be added to the vial to achieve this concentration? _____

6. The physician orders ampicillin 1 g. The label on the 2 g vial reads to reconstitute with 200 ml of normal saline. How many milliliters would contain the ordered amount? _____

7. The label on the 1 g powder of azithromycin reads to reconstitute with water to achieve a concentration of 200 mg/5 ml. How many milliliters of water should be added to achieve this concentration? _____

8. The physician orders ampicillin 0.5 g. The label on the 1 g vial of ampicillin reads to reconstitute with water to achieve a concentration of 125 mg/5 ml. How many milliliters will achieve the ordered dose? _____

9. The physician orders azithromycin 0.5 g po. The label on the vial of azithromycin reads to reconstitute with water to achieve a concentration of 200 mg/5 ml. How many milliliters will achieve the ordered dose? _____

10. The physician orders cefaclor 250 mg po. The vial of cefaclor powder for reconstitution reads to reconstitute with water to achieve a concentration of 375 mg/ 5 ml. How many milliliters will achieve the ordered dose? _____

11. The label on the 2 g vial of cefadroxil monohydrate powder reads to reconstitute with water to achieve a concentration of 125 mg/5 ml. How many milliliters of diluent should be added to achieve this concentration? _____

12. The label on the 10 g vial of cefotaxime sodium reads to reconstitute the powder with sterile water to achieve a concentration of 1 g/6 ml. How many milliliters of diluent should be added to the contents of the vial to achieve this concentration? _____

13. The physician orders cefotetan disodium 200,000 mcg IV q12h. The label on the 1 g vial of powdered cefotetan disodium reads to reconstitute with sterile water to achieve a concentration of 1 g/10 ml. How many milliliters of sterile water should be added to the powder to achieve the ordered dose? _____

14. The label on the 2 g vial of cefoxitin sodium powder reads to reconstitute with 50 ml of sterile water. This provides a concentration of _____ mg/ml.

15. The physician orders cefpodoxime proxetil 200 mg po q12h. The label on the vial of granules of cefpodoxime proxetil reads to reconstitute with distilled water to achieve a concentration of 50 mg/5 ml. The nurse should administer _____ ml of reconstituted medication to achieve ordered dose.

16. The label on the 250 mg vial of ceprozil reads to reconstitute with 5 ml of distilled water. This will provide a concentration of _____ mg/ml.

17. The physician orders ceftazidime 1 g IV. The powder for injection of cetazidime is in a vial that is labeled to reconstitute with 50 ml of normal saline for injection to achieve a concentration of 10 mg/ml. How many milliliters will be required to achieve ordered dose? _____

18. The physician orders ceftizoxime sodium 0.5 g IV q12h. The label on the vial of powder for reconstitution of ceftizoxime sodium reads to reconstitute with sterile water to achieve a concentration of 10 mg/ml The nurse should prepare to administer _____ ml to achieve the ordered dose.

19. The physician orders cefuroxime axetil 250 mg suspension. The label on the vial of cefuroxime axetil powder reads to reconstitute with distilled water to achieve a concentration of 0.12 g/ 5 ml. How many milliliters of this concentration will be needed to achieve the ordered dose? _____

20. The physician orders 500 mg cephalexin monohydrate suspension po q12h. The label on the vial of cephalexin monohydrate powder reads to reconstitute with water to achieve a concentration of 125 mg/4.5 ml. How many milliliters of reconstituted medication should the nurse administer to achieve the ordered dose? _____

21. The label of the 1 g vial of cephadine powder reads to reconstitute with 40 ml of distilled water for oral suspension. This will provide a concentration of _____ mg/ml.

22. The physician orders cephadine 0.5 g IV q6h. The label on the 2 g vial of cephadine powder reads to reconstitute with 20 ml of sterile water. How many milliliters of reconstituted medication will achieve ordered dose? _____

23. The physician orders 0.5 g chlorothiazide IV stat. The label on each of 2 vials of chlorothiazide powder reads to reconstitute with 18 ml of sterile water to 500 mg powder. The nurse should administer _____ ml to achieve ordered dose.

24. The physician orders clarithromycin 500 mg po bid. The label on the bottle of granules for oral suspension reads to reconstitute with water to achieve a concentration of 0.125 g/5 ml. The nurse should administer _____ ml of reconstituted medication to achieve ordered dose.

25. The physician orders clindamycin HCl 900 mg IV q8h. The label on the vial of clindamycin powder for injection reads to reconstitute in 5% dextrose to achieve a concentration of 10 gr/50 ml. The nurse will have to infuse _____ ml to administer the ordered dose.

26. The label on the vial of cloxacillin sodium powder reads to reconstitute with water to provide a concentration of 125 mg/5ml. The physician orders cloxacillin sodium 0.25 g po. The nurse should administer _____ ml(s).

27. A client is to receive coagulation factor VIIA intravenous bolus. It is supplied in powder that is to be reconstituted with sterile water to achieve a concentration of 4.8 mg/ 8.5 ml. The client weighs 44 kg and his dosage is based on 90 mcg/kg. The nurse should administer _____ ml(s) for the appropriate dose for this client.

28. The physician orders cyclophosphamide 550 mg IV over 90 minutes qd for 5 days. The label on the vial of cyclophosphamide powder reads to reconstitute with sterile water to achieve a concentration of 2.2 mg/ ml. The nurse should administer _____ ml(s)

29. The physician orders cefurozime sodium 750 mg IV q8h. The label on the 750 mg vial of cefuroxime sodium powder for injection reads to reconstitute with 100 ml of 5% dextrose in water. This provides a concentration of _____ mg/ml?

30. The label on the 0.5 g vial of cefaclor reads to reconstitute with water to achieve a concentration of 200 mg/ml. How many milliliters of water should be added to the vial to achieve this concentration? _____

31. The label on the 10 g vial of cefotetan disodium reads to reconstitute the powder for injection with sterile water to achieve a concentration of 1g/10 ml. How many milliliters of water should be added to the contents of the vial to achieve this concentration?

_____

32. The label on the 10 g vial of ampicillin reads to reconstitute with 50 ml of sodium chloride. This will provide a concentration of how many grams/ml? _____

33. The label on the 5 gr vial of clindamycin powder for injection reads to reconstitute in 50 ml of normal saline. This will provide a concentration of _____ mg/ml.

34. The label on the 1 g vial of cephalexin monohydrate powder reads to reconstitute with 20 ml of distilled water. This provides a concentration of _____ mg/5 ml.

35. The physician orders cefadroxil monohydrate 1000 mg po bid. The label on the vial of cefadroxil monohydrate reads to reconstitute with water to a concentration of 0.25 g/2.5 ml. How many milliliters will achieve the ordered dose? _____

36. The physician orders cefadroxil monohydrate 2 g po in 2 divided doses. The label on the vial of cefadroxil monohydrate reads to reconstitute with water to a concentration of 500 mg/5 ml. How many milliliters will achieve the ordered dose? _____

37. The physician orders cefotaxime sodium 0.5 g IM. The label on the vial of cefotaxime sodium reads to reconstitute with sterile water to achieve a concentration of 1 g/ 2 ml. How many milliliters of sterile water will achieve the ordered dose? _____

38. The physician orders cefoxitin sodium 1 g q4h IV. The vial of cefoxitin sodium powder for injection has been reconstituted with sterile water to a concentration of 20 mg/ml. How many milliliters of sterile water will be needed to achieve the ordered dose? _____

39. The label on the 1 g vial of ceftizoxime sodium powder for reconstitution reads to reconstitute with 50 ml of normal saline. This will provide a concentration of _____ mg/ml.

40. The label on the 100 mg vial of granules of cefpodoxime proxetil reads to reconstitute with 50 ml of distilled water. This will achieve a concentration of _____ mg/ml.

41. The label on the 500 mg vial of chlorothiazide powder reads to reconstitute with 18 ml of sterile water. This will provide a concentration of _____ mg/ml.

42. The physician orders clindamycin 20 gr IV. The label on the vial of clindamycin powder for injection reads to reconstitute to produce a concentration of 900 mg/50 ml. How many milliliters would be required to administer ordered dose? _____

43. The physician orders cloxacillin sodium 300 mg q6h po. The label on the vial of cloxacillin sodium reads to reconstitute with water to produce a concentration of 125 mg/5ml. The nurse should administer _____ ml(s) to administer ordered dose.

44. The label on the 0.5 g vial of acyclovir powder reads to dilute with normal saline to achieve a concentration of 3.5 mg/ml. The nurse should dilute vial with _____ ml of normal saline.

45. The physician orders 350 mg of acyclovir IV over an hour. To administer a concentration of 3 mg/ml, the nurse should administer _____ ml(s) to achieve the ordered dose.

46. The physician orders dactinomycin 1000 mcg IV. The label on the vial of dactinomycin powder reads to reconstitute with preservative-free sterile water to achieve a concentration of 0.5 mg/ml then dilute each 0.5 mg in 50 ml of sterile normal saline. How many milliliters should be used to administer ordered dose? _____

47. The label on the 20 mg vial of dantrolene sodium powder for injection reads to reconstitute with 60 ml sterile water for injection diluent. This will achieve a concentration of _____ mcg/ml.

48. The physician orders dantrolene sodium 250 mg IV to infuse over 1 hour prior to anesthesia. The label on the vial containing dantrolene sodium reads to reconstitute with sterile water to a concentration of 20 mg /6 ml. The nurse should administer _____ ml to achieve ordered dose.

49. The label on the 500 mg ampule of deferoxamine mesylate powder for injection reads to reconstitute with 2 ml of sterile water. This will provide a concentration of _____ g/ml.

50. The physician orders didanosine 200 mg po. Didanosine is supplied in a 200 mg powder for oral solution. This solution is to be reconstituted with 120 ml of water. The nurse should administer _____ ml(s) to achieve the ordered dose.

51. The label on the 25 mg vial of diltiazem HCl powder reads to reconstitute with manufacturer-supplied diluent to prepare a solution of 5 mg/ml. The nurse needs to add _____ ml of diluent to this vial to achieve the concentration on the vial.

52. The physician orders dolcusate 300 mg oral solution. The label on the 283 mg bottle of dolcusate powder reads to reconstitute with water to achieve a concentration of 30 mg/ml. How many milliliters should the nurse administer to achieve ordered dose? _____

53. The label on the 0.3 g vial of doxorubicin HCl powder reads to reconstitute each 10 mg with 5 ml of normal saline. How many milliliters of normal saline will be needed to reconstitute the vial to this concentration? _____

54. The physician orders doxycycline 100 mg IV bid. Doxycycline powder for injection is available in a 0.1 g vial, which is to be reconstituted with 10 ml of normal saline and then diluted to achieve a concentration of 0.5 mg/ml. The nurse should administer _____ ml(s) to provide ordered dose.

55. The physician orders erythromycin lactobionate IV 450 mg q6h. The label on the vial of erythromycin lactobionate powder reads to reconstitute with sterile water to a concentration of 5 mg/ml. The nurse should administer _____ ml of reconstituted medication to achieve ordered dose.

56. The label on the 0.05 g vial of ethacrynic sodium powder for injection reads to dilute with normal saline to a concentration of 1000 mcg/ml. The nurse should reconstitute with _____ ml of normal saline to the vial to produce this concentration.

57. The physician orders famotidine 20 mg po bid. The label on the 0.04 g bottle of famotidine powder reads to reconstitute with water to produce a concentration of 0.04 g/5 ml. The nurse should administer _____ ml to give ordered dose.

58. The label on the 0.5 g vial of floxuridine reads to reconstitute with 5 ml of sterile water to yield a concentration of 100 mg/ml. The nurse should reconstitute the vial with _____ ml.

59. The physician orders fluconazole 0.2 g po. The bottle of fluconazole powder has a label that reads to reconstitute with water to yeild a concentration of 50 mg/5 ml. The nurse should administer _____ ml to give ordered dose.

60. The physician orders doxycycline 100 mg po. The label on the bottle of doxycycline powder reads to reconstitute with water to prepare a concentration of 0.025 g/5 ml. The nurse should administer _____ ml to provide ordered dose.

61. The physician orders diltiazem HCl 50 mg IV. The label on the 25 mg vial of diltiazem HCl powder reads to reconstitute with normal saline to prepare a solution of 5mg/ml. How many vials will be needed to achieve the ordered dose? _____

62. The physician orders doxorubicin HCl 2.5 gr IV. The label on the 100 mg vial of doxorubicin HCl reads to reconstitute the powder in the vial with normal saline to produce a concentration of 10 mg/5 ml. After reconstituting 2 drug vials, the nurse will need to administer _____ ml to achieve ordered dose.

63. The physician orders diltiazem HCl 50 mg IV. The label on the 25 mg vial of diltiazem HCl powder reads to reconstitute with manufacturer-supplied diluent to prepare a solution of 5mg/ml. After reconstituting 2 vials, how many milliliters will be needed to achieve ordered dose? _____

64. The label on the 0.1 g vial of doxycycline hyclate powder reads to reconstitute with normal saline to produce a concentration of 0.2 mg/ml. After reconstituting two vials, the nurse would need to administer _____ ml of reconstituted drug to administer a 200 mg ordered dose.

65. The label on the bottle of dulcosate states to reconstitute 284 mg of powder with water to achieve a concentration of 4 mg/ml. How many milliliters of diluent should the nurse add to the contents of the bottle to produce this concentration? _____

66. The physician orders doxorubicin HCl 150 mg IV. The label on the 100 mg vial of doxorubicin HCl reads to reconstitute the powder in the vial with normal saline to produce a concentration of 10 mg/5 ml. How many vials will be needed to prepare ordered dose?

_____

67. The label on the 400 mg vial of erythromycin ethylsuccinate powder reads to reconstitute with water to achieve a concentration of 100 mg/2.5 ml. The nurse should reconstitute with _____ ml to achieve this concentration.

68. The physician orders ethacrynic sodium 50 mg IV. The label on the vial of ethacrynic sodium powder reads to reconstitute with normal saline to achieve a concentration of 0.001 g/ml. The nurse should administer _____ ml to produce ordered dose.

69. The label on the 0.05 g vial of doxorubicin HCl powder reads to reconstitute with normal saline to produce a concentration 10 mg/5 ml. The nurse will need to reconstitute vial with _____ ml of normal saline to achieve this concentration.

70. The physician orders erythromycin ethylsuccinate 250 mg of oral suspension. The label on the 0.4 g vial of erythromycin ethylsuccinate states to reconstitute granules with water to achieve a concentration of 100 mg/5ml. The nurse should administer _____ ml for the ordered dose.

71. The label on the 0.1 g vial of doxycycline hyclate powder reads to reconstitute with 10 ml of sterile water and then dilute with normal saline to produce a concentration of 1 mg/ml. The total amount of fluid used to achieve this concentration is _____ ml.

72. The label of the 1 g vial of erythromycin lactobionate powder reads to reconstitute with 5% dextrose in water to achieve a concentration of 1 mg/ml. The nurse would use _____ ml of 5% dextrose in water to achieve this concentration.

73. The label on the 40 mg bottle of famotidine powder reads to reconstitute with water to produce a concentration of 20 mg/4 ml. How many milliliters of diluent would be needed to reconstitute the 40 mg bottle? _____

74. The physician orders fluconazole 100 mg po. The label on the 200 mg bottle of fluconazole reads to reconstitute with water to yield 200 mg/5 ml. The nurse should administer _____ ml of the reconstituted medication.

75. The label on the vial of follitropin beta powder for injection reads to reconstitute to achieve a concentration no greater than 225 IU/0.5 ml. The nurse should reconstitute a 150 IU vial with _____ ml to produce the recommended concentration.

76. The physician orders fosfomycin tromethamine 50 gr. The packets of 3 g fosfomycin tromethamine granules have labels that read to reconstitute in 90 ml of water. The nurse should administer _____ ml to provide ordered dose.

77. The label on the 500 mg vial of ganciclovir sodium powder for injection reads to reconstitute in 10 ml of sterile water to achieve a concentration of 50 mg/ml and then further dilute to yield a concentration of 10 mg/ml. To produce a 10 mg/ml concentration for a 500 mg vial, the nurse should use _____ ml.

78. The physician orders hydrocortisone sodium succinate 120 mg IV q12h. The 100 mg vials containing the hydrocortisone sodium succinate have labels that read to reconstitute each vial with 2 ml of bacteriostatic water for injection. After reconstituting 2 vials, the nurse should administer _____ ml to deliver ordered dose.

79. The physician orders immune globulin IV (human) 24 g IV once a month. The label on the 6 g vial of immune globulin IV (human) powder for injection reads to reconstitute to achieve a concentration of 50 mg/ml. After reconstituting 2 vials, the nurse should administer _____ ml to provide ordered dose.

80. The label on the 100 mg vial of infliximab powder for injection reads to reconstitute with sterile water to achieve a concentration of 10 mg/ml. The vial should be reconstituted with _____ ml of diluent.

81. The physician orders infliximab 315 mg IV. The vial of infliximab powder for injection should be reconstituted with sterile water to yield a concentration of 10 mg/ml. The nurse should administer _____ ml to provide ordered dose.

82. The physician orders lepirudin 28.8 mg IV. The label on the 50 mg vial of lipirudin states to reconstitute with normal saline to yield a concentration of 5mg/ml. The nurse should administer _____ ml of the reconstituted agent to give ordered dose.

83. The physician orders leuprolide acetate ½ gr SC qd. The label on the 15 mg vial of leuprolide acetate powder for injection reads to reconstitute with sterile water to yield a concentration of 7.5 mg/0.1 ml. The nurse should administer _____ ml to provide ordered dose.

84. The label on the 3 g packet of fosfomycin tromethamine granules reads to reconstitute in 120 ml of water. This will provide a concentration of _____ mg/ml.

85. The physician orders ganciclovir sodium 275 mg IV. The 500 mg vial of gancyclovir sodium requires reconstitution with sterile water to a concentration of 10 mg/ml. The nurse should administer _____ ml to achieve ordered dose.

86. The physician orders hydrocortisone sodium succinate 80 mg IV q8h. The label on the 200 mg vial of hydrocortisone reads to reconstitute with 2 ml of sterile water for injection. The nurse should administer _____ ml to achieve ordered dose.

87. The label on the 3 g vial of immune globulin IV (human) powder for injection reads to reconstitute to yield a concentration of 0.05g/ml. The nurse should reconstitute the vial with _____ ml to produce the labeled concentration.

88. The label on the ¼ gr vial of leuprolide powder for injection reads to reconstitute with sterile water to yield a concentration of 7.5 mg/0.1 ml. To reconstitute this vial, the nurse should use _____ ml of diluent.

89. The physician orders 1 g of meropenem IV q8h. The labels on the 1000 mg vials of meropenem powder for injection read to reconstitute with sterile water to a concentration of 50 mg/ml. The nurse should reconstitute using _____ ml to administer ordered dose.

90. The label on the 5.8 mg vial of somatrem/somatropin powder for injection states to reconstitute with bacteriostatic water to yield a concentration of 2.9 mg/0.5 ml. The nurse should use _____ ml to reconstitute this vial.

91. The label on the 2g vial of spectinomycin HCl powder for injection states to reconstitute to achieve a concentration of 750 mg/ml. The nurse should use _____ ml of diluent to reconstitute this vial.

92. The physician orders 250 mg po of tolbutamide sodium. The label on the 1 g vial of tolbutamide sodium powder reads to reconstitute with water to yield a concentration of 0.25 g/5 ml. The nurse reconstitutes the vial with _____ ml to create concentration and then administers _____ ml to give ordered dose.

93. The physician orders 500 mcg of somatrem/somatropin SC. The label on the 1.5 mg vial of somatrem/somatropin powder for injection reads to reconstitute with sterile water to yield concentration of 1.5 mg/3 ml. The nurse should administer _____ ml of reconstituted drug for ordered dose.

94. The label on the vial of 250,000 units of urokinase reads to reconstitute to a concentration of 1,500 u/ml. To reconstitute the vial, _____ ml of diluent must be used.

95. The physician orders 2g vancomycin HCl po in 4 divided doses per day. The label on the 2 g bottle of vancomycin HCl powder for reconstitution reads to use sterile water to yield a concentration of 500 mg/6 ml. The nurse should add _____ ml of diluent to administer each dose.

96. The physician orders 125 mg of vacomycin HCl po tid. The label on the 0.25 g bottle of vancomycin HCl powder reads to reconstitute with sterile water to achieve a concentration of 50 mg/ml. The nurse should administer _____ ml to give ordered dose.

97. The label on the vial of 1/12 gr of warfarin sodium reads to reconstitute with sterile water to yield a concentration of 1 mg/ml. The nurse should use _____ ml of diluent to reconstitute this vial.

98. The physician orders 5 mg of warfarin sodium IV. The label on the vial of warfarin sodium reads to reconstitute with sterile water to yield a concentration of 1 mg/ml. The nurse should administer _____ ml to give ordered dose.

99. The physician orders cephalexin monohydrate 500 mg po. The powder for reconstitution of cephalexin monohydrate is to be reconstituted with water to a concentration of 0.25 g/5 ml. The nurse should use _____ ml to achieve ordered dose.

100. The label on a 1 g vial of a powdered medication reads to reconstitute to achieve a concentration of 125 mg/5 ml. The nurse should add _____ ml to the vial to yield the accepted concentration.

Answers for Unit V

1. 2 ml
2. 0.45 ml
3. 2.5 ml
4. 40 ml
5. 200 ml
6. 100 ml
7. 25 ml
8. 20 ml
9. 12.5 ml
10. 3.3 ml
11. 80 ml
12. 60 ml
13. 2 ml
14. 40 mg/ml
15. 20 ml
16. 50 mg/ml
17. 100 ml
18. 50 ml
19. 10.4 ml
20. 18 ml
21. 25 mg/ml
22. 5 ml
23. 18 ml
24. 20 ml
25. 75 ml
26. 10 ml
27. 7 ml
28. 250 ml
29. 7.5 mg/ml
30. 2.5 ml
31. 100 ml
32. 0.2 g/ml
33. 6 mg/ml
34. 250 mg/5 ml
35. 10 ml
36. 10 ml
37. 1 ml
38. 50 ml
39. 20 mg/ml
40. 2 mg/ml
41. 27.8 mg/ml
42. 66.7 ml or 67 ml
43. 12 ml
44. 142.9 or 143 ml
45. 116.7 or 117 ml
46. 100 ml
47. 333 mcg/ml
48. 75 ml
49. 0.25 g/ml
50. 120 ml
51. 5 ml
52. 10 ml
53. 150 ml
54. 200 ml

55. 90 ml

56. 50 ml

57. 2.5 ml

58. 5 ml

59. 20 ml

60. 20 ml

61. 2 vials

62. 75 ml

63. 10 ml

64. 1000 ml

65. 71 ml

66. 2 vials of which 1½ vials will be administered after reconstitution

67. 10 ml

68. 50 ml

69. 25 ml

70. 12.5 ml

71. 100 ml

72. 1000 ml

73. 8 ml

74. 2.5 ml

75. 0.33 ml

76. 90 ml

77. 50 ml

78. 2.4 ml

79. 480 ml

80. 10 ml

81. 31.5 ml

82. 5.8 ml

83. 0.4 ml

84. 25 ml

85. 27.5 ml

86. 0.8 ml

87. 60 ml

88. 0.2 ml

89. 20 ml

90. 1 ml

91. 2.7 ml

92. 20 ml and 5 ml

93. 1 ml

94. 166.7 ml or 167 ml

95. 6 ml

96. 2.5 ml

97. 5 ml

98. 5 ml

99. 10 ml

100. 40 ml

Intravenous Infusions—
Calculating Infusion Rates

Fill in the hourly rates for the following orders.

1. Doctor's order: 1000 ml D_5W to infuse over 8 hours
   Hourly rate: _____

2. Doctor's order: 500 ml D_5NS to infuse over 6 hours
   Hourly rate: _____

3. Doctor's order: 250 ml NS to infuse over 2 hours
   Hourly rate: _____

4. Doctor's order: 2000 ml $D_5W/\frac{1}{2}$ NS to infuse over 10 hours
   Hourly rate: _____

5. Doctor's order: 1500 ml $D_5W/\frac{1}{4}$ NS to infuse over 12 hours
   Hourly rate: _____

6. Doctor's order: 250 ml of vancomycin 500 mg to infuse over 90 minutes
   Hourly rate: _____

7. Doctor's order: 3000 ml D$_5$W/NS to infuse over 24 hours
   Hourly rate: _____

8. Doctor's order: 90 ml D$_5$W/½ NS to infuse over 2 hours
   Hourly rate: _____

9. Doctor's order: 750 ml NS to infuse over 8 hours
   Hourly rate: _____

10. Doctor's order: 50 ml cefazolin sodium 1 gram to infuse over 15 minutes.
    Hourly rate: _____

11. Doctor's order: 100 ml gentamycin 80 mg to infuse over 30 minutes.
    Hourly rate: _____

12. Doctor's order: 25 ml diphenhydramine 25 mg to infuse over 30 minutes.
    Hourly rate: _____

13. Doctor's order: 250 ml of vancomycin 500 mg to infuse over 60 minutes
    Hourly rate: _____

14. Doctor's order: 1000 ml of D_5W/NS to infuse over 10 hours
    Hourly rate: _____

15. Doctor's order: 500 ml of NS to infuse over 4 hours
    Hourly rate: _____

16. Doctor's order: 275 ml of D_5W to infuse over 3 hours
    Hourly rate: _____

17. Doctor's order: 3000 ml of lactated Ringer's to infuse over 12 hours
    Hourly rate: _____

18. Doctor's order: 150 ml of NS to infuse over 2 hours
    Hourly rate: _____

19. Doctor's order: 125 ml of D_{10}W to infuse over 60 minutes
    Hourly rate: _____

20. Doctor's order: 1000 ml D_5W/½ NS to infuse over 6 hours
    Hourly rate: _____

21. Doctor's order: 100 ml ampicillin sodium 500 mg to infuse over 40 minutes
    Hourly rate: _____

22. Doctor's order: 760 ml D_5W to infuse over 4 hours
    Hourly rate: _____

23. Doctor's order: 200 ml 0.9% normal saline to infuse over 2 hours
    Hourly rate: _____

24. Doctor's order: 350 ml lactated Ringer's to infuse over 5 hours
    Hourly rate: _____

25. Doctor's order: 250 ml lactated Ringer's to infuse over 5 hours
    Hourly rate: _____

26. Doctor's order: 250 ml D_5W/½ NS with 20 mEq KCl to infuse over 10 hours
    Hourly rate: _____

27. Doctor's order: Two 320 ml packed red blood cells (blood) to infuse over 4 hours
    Hourly rate: _____

28. Doctor's order: 320 ml packed red blood cells (blood) to infuse over 4 hours
Hourly rate: _____

29. Doctor's order: 2700 ml of D_5W to infuse over 24 hours
Hourly rate: _____

30. Doctor's order: 1250 ml of D_5W/¼ NS to infuse over 24 hours
Hourly rate: _____

31. Doctor's order: 300 ml of normal saline to infuse over 30 hours
Hourly rate: _____

32. Doctor's order: 1200 ml of D_5W to infuse over 6 hours
Hourly rate: _____

33. Doctor's order: 1500 ml of lactated Ringer's to infuse over 10 hours
Hourly rate: _____

34. Doctor's order: 2000 ml of NS to infuse over 8 hours
Hourly rate: _____

35. Doctor's order: 600 ml of normal saline to infuse over 10 hours
    Hourly rate: _____

36. Doctor's order: 2000 ml of D_5W to infuse over 12 hours
    Hourly rate: _____

37. Doctor's order: 0.5 L of D_5/½ normal saline with 20 mEq potassium chloride to infuse over 10 hours
    Hourly rate: _____

38. Doctor's order: 1200 ml NS to infuse over 8 hours
    Hourly rate: _____

39. Doctor's order: 650 ml of normal saline to infuse over 10 hours
    Hourly rate: _____

40. Doctor's order: 1500 ml of D_5W to infuse over 24 hours
    Hourly rate: _____

41. Doctor's order: 0.3 L of D_5W to infuse over 10 hours
    Hourly rate: _____

42. Doctor's order: 1200 ml D_5W/NS to infuse over 12 hours
    Hourly rate: _____

43. Doctor's order: 1500 ml to NS to infuse over 15 hours
    Hourly rate: _____

44. Doctor's order: 200 ml of NS to infuse over 2 hours
    Hourly rate: _____

45. Doctor's order: 5 L of D_5W/½ NS to infuse over 36 hours
    Hourly rate: _____

46. Doctor's order: 2 L of NS to infuse over 18 hours
    Hourly rate: _____

47. Doctor's order: 0.5 L of NS to infuse over 2 hours
    Hourly rate: _____

48. Doctor's order: 750 ml of D_5W/¼ NS to infuse over 6 hours
    Hourly rate: _____

49. Doctor's order: 0.75 L of lactated Ringer's to infuse over 4 hours
    Hourly rate: _____

50. Doctor's order: 25 ml of ondansetron to infuse over 15 minutes
    Hourly rate: _____

51. Doctor's order: 4000 ml of $D_5W/\frac{1}{2}$ NS to infuse over 40 hours
    Hourly rate: _____

52. Doctor's order: 25 ml of diphenhydramine to infuse over 20 minutes.
    Hourly rate: _____

53. Doctor's order: 250 ml of vancomycin to infuse over 75 minutes
    Hourly rate: _____

54. Doctor's order: 50 ml of cefoxitin sodium 1 g to infuse over 30 minutes
    Hourly rate: _____

55. Doctor's order: 100 ml of sodium chloride over infuse over 15 minutes
    Hourly rate: _____

56. Doctor's order: 320 ml of packed red blood cells (blood) to infuse over 3 hours
    Hourly rate: _____

57. Doctor's order: 60 ml D_5W to infuse over 15 minutes
    Hourly rate: _____

58. Doctor's order: 50 ml of cephapirin sodium 500 mg to infuse over 40 minutes
    Hourly rate: _____

59. Doctor's order: 50 ml of ceftriaxone sodium 1 g to infuse over 45 minutes
    Hourly rate: _____

60. Doctor's order: 100 ml of sodium chloride to infuse over 20 minutes
    Hourly rate: _____

61. Doctor's order: 100 ml of sodium chloride to infuse over 45 minutes
    Hourly rate: _____

62. Doctor's order: 160 ml of packed red blood cells (blood) to infuse over 4 hours
    Hourly rate: _____

63. Doctor's order: 200 ml of packed red blood cells (blood) to infuse over 3 hours
    Hourly rate: _____

64. Doctor's order: 400 ml of normal saline to infuse over 2 hours
    Hourly rate: _____

65. Doctor's order: 150 ml of sodium chloride to infuse over 1½ hours
    Hourly rate: _____

66. Doctor's order: 70 ml of $D_{10}W$ to infuse over 2 hours
    Hourly rate: _____

67. Doctor's order: 250 ml of $D_{10}W$ to infuse over 5 hours
    Hourly rate: _____

68. Doctor's order: 300 ml of lactated Ringer's to infuse over 3 hours
    Hourly rate: _____

69. Doctor's order: 350 ml of D_5W to infuse over 3 hours
    Hourly rate: _____

70. Doctor's order: 5 L of lactated Ringer's to infuse over 24 hours
    Hourly rate: _____

71. Doctor's order: 350 ml of ¼ normal saline to infuse over 4 hours
    Hourly rate: _____

72. Doctor's order: 5000 ml of D_5/½ normal saline to infuse over 48 hours
    Hourly rate: _____

73. Doctor's order: 350 ml of D_5W with 40 mEq of sodium bicarbonate to infuse over
    5 hours
    Hourly rate: _____

74. Doctor's order: 150 ml of D_5W to infuse over 2½ hours
    Hourly rate: _____

75. Doctor's order: 4.5L of lactated Ringer's to infuse over 48 hours
    Hourly rate: _____

76. Doctor's order: 300 ml of $D_{10}W$ to infuse over 5 hours
    Hourly rate: _____

77. Doctor's order: 1566 ml of total parenteral nutrition (TPN) to infuse over 18 hours
    Hourly rate: _____

78. Doctor's order: 1656 of total parenteral nutrition (TPN) to infuse over 24 hours
    Hourly rate: _____

79. Doctor's order: 72 ml of intralipids to infuse over 18 hours
    Hourly rate: _____

80. Doctor's order: 240 ml of D_5W to infuse over 90 minutes
    Hourly rate: _____

81. Doctor's order: 350 ml of D_5W to infuse over 5 hours
    Hourly rate: _____

82. Doctor's order: 180 ml of intralipids to infuse over 18 hours
    Hourly rate: _____

83. Doctor's order: 3200 ml of $D_5/\frac{1}{4}$ normal saline to infuse over 24 hours
    Hourly rate: _____

84. Doctor's order: 350 ml of $D_{10}W$ to infuse over 2 hours
    Hourly rate: _____

85. Doctor's order: 270 ml of $D_{10}W$ to infuse over 3 hours
    Hourly rate: _____

86. Doctor's order: 350 ml of normal saline to infuse over 7 hours
    Hourly rate: _____

87. Doctor's order: 300 ml of ½ normal saline to infuse over 10 hours
    Hourly rate: _____

88. Doctor's order: 420 ml of ¼ normal saline to infuse over 7 hours
    Hourly rate: _____

89. Doctor's order: 4L of D_5/½ normal saline with 20 mEq potassium chloride to infuse over 48 hours
    Hourly rate: _____

90. Doctor's order: 576 ml of TPN to infuse over 24 hours
    Hourly rate: _____

91. Doctor's order: 30 ml of ondansetron to infuse over 15 minutes
    Hourly rate: _____

92. Doctor's order: 0.4 L of D_5W/normal saline to infuse over 2 hours
    Hourly rate: _____

93. Doctor's order: 500 ml of D_5W with 20 mEq of potassium chloride to infuse over 15 hours
    Hourly rate: _____

94. Doctor's order: 750 ml of D_5W to infuse over 10 hours
    Hourly rate: _____

95. Doctor's order: 1 L of D_5W/normal saline to infuse over 4 hours
    Hourly rate: _____

96. Doctor's order: 1000 ml of lactated Ringer's to infuse over 20 hours
    Hourly rate: _____

97. Doctor's order: 1.5 L of D_5W/¼ normal saline to infuse over 10 hours
    Hourly rate: _____

98. Doctor's order: 2000 ml of normal saline to infuse over 24 hours
    Hourly rate: _____

99. Doctor's order: 1512 ml of TPN to infuse over 36 hours
    Hourly rate: _____

100. Doctor's order: 162 ml of intralipids to infuse over 18 hours
    Hourly rate: _____

101. Doctor's order: 2750 ml of D_5/½ normal saline to infuse over 24 hours
    Hourly rate: _____

102. Doctor's order: 0.8 L of normal saline to infuse over 10 hours
    Hourly rate: _____

103. Doctor's order: 1000 ml of D_5/½ normal saline with 20 mEq of potassium chloride over 12 hours
    Hourly rate: _____

104. Doctor's order: 500 ml of vancomycin 1 g to infuse over 2 hours
    Hourly rate: _____

Answers for Unit VI

1. 125 ml/hr
2. 83 ml/hr
3. 125 ml/hr
4. 200 ml/hr
5. 125 ml/hr
6. 167 ml/hr
7. 125 ml/hr
8. 45 ml/hr
9. 94 ml/hr
10. 200 ml/hr
11. 200 ml/hr
12. 50 ml/hr
13. 250 ml/hr
14. 100 ml/hr
15. 125 ml/hr
16. 92 ml/hr
17. 250 ml/hr
18. 75 ml/hr
19. 125 ml/hr
20. 167 ml/hr
21. 150 ml/hr
22. 190 ml/hr
23. 100 ml/hr
24. 70 ml/hr
25. 50 ml/hr
26. 25 ml/hr
27. 160 ml/hr
28. 80 ml/hr
29. 112.5 or 113 ml/hr
30. 52 ml/hr
31. 10 ml/hr
32. 200 ml/hr
33. 150 ml/hr
34. 250 ml/hr
35. 60 ml/hr
36. 167 ml/hr
37. 50 ml/hr
38. 150 ml/hr
39. 65 ml/hr
40. 62.5 or 63 ml/hr
41. 30 ml/hr
42. 100 ml/hr
43. 100 ml/hr
44. 100 ml/hr
45. 139 ml/hr
46. 111 ml/hr
47. 250 ml/hr
48. 125 ml/hr
49. 187.5 or 188 ml/hr
50. 100 ml/hr
51. 100 ml/hr
52. 75 ml/hr
53. 200 ml/hr
54. 100 ml/hr

55. 400 ml/hr	80. 160 ml/hr
56. 107 ml/hr	81. 70 ml/hr
57. 240 ml/hr	82. 10 ml/hr
58. 75 ml/hr	83. 133 ml/hr
59. 67 ml/hr	84. 175 ml/hr
60. 300 ml/hr	85. 90 ml/hr
61. 133 ml/hr	86. 50 ml/hr
62. 40 ml/hr	87. 30 ml/hr
63. 67 ml/hr	88. 60 ml/hr
64. 200 ml/hr	89. 83 ml/hr
65. 100 ml/hr	90. 24 ml/hr
66. 35 ml/hr	91. 120 ml/hr
67. 50 ml/hr	92. 200 ml/hr
68. 100 ml/hr	93. 33 ml/hr
69. 117 ml/hr	94. 75 ml/hr
70. 208 ml/hr	95. 250 ml/hr
71. 87.5 or 88 ml/hr	96. 50 ml/hr
72. 104 ml/hr	97. 150 ml/hr
73. 70 ml/hr	98. 83 ml/hr
74. 60 ml/hr	99. 42 ml/hr
75. 94 ml/hr	100. 9 ml/hr
76. 60 ml/hr	101. 115 ml/hr
77. 87 ml/hr	102. 80 ml/hr
78. 69 ml/hr	103. 83 ml/hr
79. 4 ml/hr	104. 250 ml/hr

Intravenous Infusions—Calculating Flow Rates Using Drip Factors

NOTE: *Because drops (gtt) are only delivered in whole numbers, answers to these calculations must be rounded using the standard rounding rule: 0.1–0.4 round down to the whole number (e.g., 83.3 gtt = 83 gtt) and 0.5–0.9 round up to the next whole number (e.g., 83.6 gtt = 84 gtt.)*

1. Doctor's order: 1000 ml D_5W to infuse over 8 hours
   Drip factor: 20 gtt/ml
   _____ gtt/min

2. Doctor's order: 500 ml D_5NS to infuse over 6 hours
   Drip factor: 60 gtt/ml
   _____ gtt/min

3. Doctor's order: 250 ml NS to infuse over 2 hours
   Drip factor: 10 gtt/ml
   _____ gtt/min

4. Doctor's order: 2000 ml $D_5W/½$ NS to infuse over 10 hours
   Drip factor: 15 gtt/ml
   _____ gtt/min

5. Doctor's order: 1500 ml D_5W/¼ NS to infuse over 12 hours
   Drip factor: 10 gtt/ml
   _____ gtt/min

6. Doctor's order: 3000 ml D_5W/NS to infuse over 24 hours
   Drip factor: 20 gtt/ml
   _____ gtt/min

7. Doctor's order: 1000 ml D_5W/½ NS to infuse over 8 hours
   Drip factor: 10 gtt/ml
   _____ gtt/min

8. Doctor's order: 750 ml NS to infuse over 8 hours
   Drip factor: 60 gtt/ml
   _____ gtt/min

9. Doctor's order: 50 ml cefazolin sodium 1 gram to infuse over 15 minutes
   Drip factor: 10 gtt/ml
   _____ gtt/min

10. Doctor's order: 100 ml gentamycin 80 mg to infuse over 30 minutes
    Drip factor: 20 gtt/ml
    _____ gtt/min

11. Doctor's order: 25 ml diphenhydramine 25 mg to infuse over 30 minutes
    Drip factor: 15 gtt/ml
    _____ gtt/min

12. Doctor's order: 1000 ml of D_5W/NS to infuse over 10 hours
    Drip factor: 20 gtt/ml
    _____ gtt/min

13. Doctor's order: 500 ml of NS to infuse over 4 hours
    Drip factor: 10 gtt/ml
    _____ gtt/min

14. Doctor's order: 250 ml of D_5W to infuse over 3 hours
    Drip factor: 20 gtt/ml
    _____ gtt/min

15. Doctor's order: 3000 ml of lactated Ringer's to infuse over 12 hours
    Drip factor: 15 gtt/ml
    _____ gtt/min

16. Doctor's order: 150 ml of NS to infuse over 4 hours
    Drip factor: 60 gtt/ml
    _____ gtt/min

17. Doctor's order: 125 ml of $D_{10}W$ to infuse over 60 minutes
    Drip factor: 15 gtt/ml
    _____ gtt/min

18. Doctor's order: 1000 ml $D_5W/\frac{1}{2}$ NS to infuse over 6 hours
    Drip factor: 20 gtt/ml
    _____ gtt/min

19. Doctor's order: 100 ml ampicillin sodium 500 mg to infuse over 40 min
Drip factor: 20 gtt/ml
_____ gtt/min

20. Doctor's order: 750 ml D_5W to infuse over 4 hours
Drip factor: 10 gtt/ml
_____ gtt/min

21. Doctor's order: 200 ml 0.9% normal saline to infuse over 2 hours
Drip factor: 20 gtt/ml
_____ gtt/min

22. Doctor's order: 3000 ml lactated Ringer's to infuse over 24 hours
Drip factor: 10 gtt/ml
_____ gtt/min

23. Doctor's order: 250 ml lactated Ringer's to infuse over 5 hours
Drip factor: 60 gtt/ml
_____ gtt/min

24. Doctor's order: D_5W/½ NS with 20 mEq KCl to infuse at 25 ml/hr
Drip factor: 60 gtt/ml
_____ gtt/min

25. Doctor's order: Two 320 ml packed red blood cells (blood) to infuse over 4 hours
Drip factor: 15 gtt/ml
_____ gtt/min

26. Doctor's order: 320 ml packed red blood cells (blood) to infuse over 4 hours
    Drip factor: 20 gtt/ml
    _____ gtt/min

27. Doctor's order: 2700 ml of D_5W to infuse over 24 hours
    Drip factor: 10 gtt/ml
    _____ gtt/min

28. Doctor's order: 1250 ml of D_5W/¼ NS to infuse over 24 hours
    Drip factor: 60 gtt/ml
    _____ gtt/min

29. Doctor's order: 75 ml/hr of NS
    Drip factor: 60 gtt/ml
    _____ gtt/min

30. Doctor's order: 1200 ml of D_5W to infuse over 6 hours
    Drip factor: 20 gtt/ml
    _____ gtt/min

31. Doctor's order: 1500 ml of lactated Ringer's to infuse over 10 hours
    Drip factor: 10 gtt/ml
    _____ gtt/min

32. Doctor's order: 2000 ml of NS to infuse over 10 hours
    Drip factor: 10 gtt/ml
    _____ gtt/min

33. Doctor's order: 60 ml/hr of NS
    Drip factor: 60 gtt/ml
    _____ gtt/min

34. Doctor's order: 2000 ml of D_5W to infuse over 10 hours
    Drip factor: 20 gtt/ml
    _____ gtt/min

35. Doctor's order: 50 ml/hr of NS
    Drip factor: 60 gtt/ml
    _____ gtt/min

36. Doctor's order: 1200 ml NS to infuse over 6 hours
    Drip factor: 10 gtt/ml
    _____ gtt/min

37. Doctor's order: 65 ml/hr of NS
    Drip factor: 60 gtt/ml
    _____ gtt/min

38. Doctor's order: 1500 ml of D_5W to infuse over 10 hours
    Drip factor: 15 gtt/ml
    _____ gtt/min

39. Doctor's order: 30 ml/hr of D_5W
    Drip factor: 60 gtt/ml
    _____ gtt/min

40. Doctor's order: 1200 ml D$_5$W/NS to infuse over 6 hours
    Drip factor: 15 gtt/ml
    _____ gtt/min

41. Doctor's order: 1500 ml to NS to infuse over 10 hours
    Drip factor: 20 gtt/ml
    _____ gtt/min

42. Doctor's order: 200 ml of NS to infuse over 2 hours
    Drip factor: 15 gtt/ml
    _____ gtt/min

43. Doctor's order: 5 L of D$_5$W/½ NS to infuse over 36 hours
    Drip factor: 10 gtt/ml
    _____ gtt/min

44. Doctor's order: 2 L of NS to infuse over 24 hours
    Drip factor: 10 gtt/ml
    _____ gtt/min

45. Doctor's order: 0.5 L of NS to infuse over 2 hours
    Drip factor: 15 gtt/ml
    _____ gtt/min

46. Doctor's order: 750 ml of D$_5$W/¼ NS to infuse over 6 hours
    Drip factor: 15 gtt/ml
    _____ gtt/min

47. Doctor's order: 0.75 L of lactated Ringer's to infuse over 4 hours
    Drip factor: 15 gtt/ml
    _____ gtt/min

48. Doctor's order: 25 ml of ondansetron to infuse over 15 minutes
    Drip factor: 10 gtt/ml
    _____ gtt/min

49. Doctor's order: 4000 ml of $D_5W/\frac{1}{2}$ NS to infuse over 40 hours
    Drip factor: 15 gtt/ml
    _____ gtt/min

50. Doctor's order: 25 ml of diphenhydramine to infuse over 20 minutes
    Drip factor: 10 gtt/ml
    _____ gtt/min

51. Doctor's order: 250 ml of vancomycin to infuse over 1½ hours
    Drip factor: 10 gtt/ml
    _____ gtt/min

52. Doctor's order: 50 ml of cefoxitin sodium 1 g to infuse over 30 minutes
    Drip factor: 10 gtt/ml
    _____ gtt/min

53. Doctor's order: 100 ml of sodium chloride to infuse over 15 minutes
    Drip factor: 15 gtt/ml
    _____ gtt/min

54. Doctor's order: 320 ml of packed red blood cells (blood) to infuse over 3 hours
    Drip factor: 20 gtt/ml
    _____ gtt/min

55. Doctor's order: 60 ml D_5W to infuse over 15 minutes
    Drip factor: 10 gtt/ml
    _____ gtt/min

56. Doctor's order: 50 ml of cephapirin sodium 500 mg to infuse over 30 minutes
    Drip factor: 15 gtt/ml
    _____ gtt/min

57. Doctor's order: 50 ml of ceftriaxone sodium 1 g to infuse over 30 minutes
    Drip factor: 20 gtt/ml
    _____ gtt/min

58. Doctor's order: 100 ml of sodium chloride to infuse over 15 minutes
    Drip factor: 10 gtt/ml
    _____ gtt/min

59. Doctor's order: 100 ml of sodium chloride to infuse over 45 minutes
    Drip factor: 20 gtt/ml
    _____ gtt/min

60. Doctor's order: 160 ml of packed red blood cells (blood) to infuse over 4 hours
    Drip factor: 20 gtt/ml
    _____ gtt/min

61. Doctor's order: 200 ml of packed red blood cells (blood) to infuse over 3 hours
    Drip factor: 10 gtt/ml
    _____ gtt/min

62. Doctor's order: Normal saline to infuse at 40 ml/hr
    Drip factor: 60 gtt/ml
    _____ gtt/min

63. Doctor's order: 150 ml of sodium chloride to infuse over 1½ hours
    Drip factor: 10 gtt/ml
    _____ gtt/min

64. Doctor's order: 70 ml of $D_{10}W$ to infuse over 2 hours
    Drip factor: 20 gtt/ml
    _____ gtt/min

65. Doctor's order: 250 ml of $D_{10}W$ to infuse over 2 hours
    Drip factor: 15 gtt/ml
    _____ gtt/min

66. Doctor's order: 300 ml of lactated Ringer's to infuse over 3 hours
    Drip factor: 10 gtt/ml
    _____ gtt/min

67. Doctor's order: 350 ml of D_5W to infuse over 3 hours
    Drip factor: 10 gtt/ml
    _____ gtt/min

68. Doctor's order: 5 L of lactated Ringer's to infuse over 24 hours
    Drip factor: 10 gtt/ml
    _____ gtt/min

69. Doctor's order: 350 ml of ¼ normal saline to infuse over 4 hours
    Drip factor: 10 gtt/ml
    _____ gtt/min

70. Doctor's order: 5000 ml of D_5/½ normal saline to infuse over 48 hours
    Drip factor: 15 gtt/ml
    _____ gtt/min

71. Doctor's order: 350 ml of D_5W with 40 mEq of sodium bicarbonate to infuse over 4 hours
    Drip factor: 15 gtt/ml
    _____ gtt/min

72. Doctor's order: 150 ml of D_5W to infuse over 1½ hours
    Drip factor: 15 gtt/ml
    _____ gtt/min

73. Doctor's order: 5 L of lactated Ringer's to infuse over 48 hours
    Drip factor: 20 gtt/ml
    _____ gtt/min

74. Doctor's order: 300 ml of D_{10}W to infuse over 5 hours
    Drip factor: 60 gtt/ml
    _____ gtt/min

75. Doctor's order: 150 ml of $D_{10}W$ to infuse over 1½ hours
    Drip factor: 20 gtt/ml
    _____ gtt/min

76. Doctor's order: 5 L of D_5W with 20 mEq of potassium to infuse over 48 hours
    Drip factor: 10 gtt/ml
    _____ gtt/min

77. Doctor's order: 300 ml of ½ normal saline to infuse over 3 hours
    Drip factor: 15 gtt/ml
    _____ gtt/min

78. Doctor's order: 250 ml of D_5W to infuse over 2 hours
    Drip factor: 20 gtt/ml
    _____ gtt/min

79. Doctor's order: 350 ml of D_5W to infuse over 3 hours
    Drip factor: 20 gtt/ml
    _____ gtt/min

80. Doctor's order: 300 ml of D_5/½ normal saline to infuse over 3 hours
    Drip factor: 20 gtt/ml
    _____ gtt/min

81. Doctor's order: 5000 ml of D_5/¼ normal saline to infuse over 45 hours
    Drip factor: 20 gtt/ml
    _____ gtt/min

82. Doctor's order: 350 ml of $D_{10}W$ to infuse over 2 hours
    Drip factor: 15 gtt/ml
    _____ gtt/min

83. Doctor's order: 300 ml of D_5W to infuse over 6 hours
    Drip factor: 60 gtt/ml
    _____ gtt/min

84. Doctor's order: 350 ml of normal saline to infuse over 2 hours
    Drip factor: 10 gtt/ml
    _____ gtt/min

85. Doctor's order: 300 ml of ½ normal saline to infuse over 4 hours
    Drip factor: 20 gtt/ml
    _____ gtt/min

86. Doctor's order: 350 ml of ¼ normal saline to infuse over 7 hours
    Drip factor: 60 gtt/ml
    _____ gtt/min

87. Doctor's order: 4L of D_5/½ normal saline with 20 mEq potassium chloride to infuse
    over 48 hours
    Drip factor: 15 gtt/ml
    _____ gtt/min

88. Doctor's order: 3000 ml of normal saline to infuse over 24 hours
    Drip factor: 10 gtt/ml
    _____ gtt/min

89. Doctor's order: 3 L of D_5W to infuse over 24 hours
    Drip factor: 15 gtt/ml
    _____ gtt/min

90. Doctor's order: 0.4 L of D_5W/normal saline to infuse over 2 hours
    Drip factor: 10 gtt/ml
    _____ gtt/min

91. Doctor's order: 500 ml of D_5W with 20 mEq of potassium chloride to infuse over 3 hours
    Drip factor: 20 gtt/ml
    _____ gtt/min

92. Doctor's order: 750 ml of D_5W to infuse over 10 hours
    Drip factor: 60 gtt/ml
    _____ gtt/min

93. Doctor's order: 1 L of D_5W/normal saline to infuse over 4 hours
    Drip factor: 10 gtt/ml
    _____ gtt/min

94. Doctor's order: 1000 ml of lactated Ringer's to infuse over 8 hours
    Drip factor: 15 gtt/ml
    _____ gtt/min

95. Doctor's order: 1500 ml of D_5W/¼ normal saline to infuse over 10 hours
    Drip factor: 20 gtt/ml
    _____ gtt/min

96. Doctor's order: 2000 ml of normal saline to infuse over 24 hours
    Drip factor: 60 gtt/ml
    _____ gtt/min

97. Doctor's order: 2 L of D_5W to infuse in 12 hours
    Drip factor: 10 gtt/ml
    _____ gtt/min

98. Doctor's order: 3 L of lactated Ringer's to infuse over 24 hours
    Drip factor: 10 gtt/ml
    _____ gtt/min

99. Doctor's order: 4000 ml of D_5/½ normal saline to infuse over 40 hours
    Drip factor: 15 gtt/ml
    _____ gtt/min

100. Doctor's order: 0.75 L of normal saline to infuse over 6 hours
     Drip factor: 60 gtt/ml
     _____ gtt/min

101. Doctor's order: 1000 ml of D_5/½ normal saline with 20 mEq of potassium chloride over
     10 hours
     Drip factor: 10 gtt/ml
     _____ gtt/min

Answers for Unit VII

1.	42 gtt/min	28.	52 gtt/min
2.	83 gtt/min	29.	75 gtt/min
3.	21 gtt/min	30.	67 gtt/min
4.	50 gtt/min	31.	25 gtt/min
5.	21 gtt/min	32.	33 gtt/min
6.	42 gtt/min	33.	60 gtt/min
7.	21 gtt/min	34.	67 gtt/min
8.	94 gtt/min	35.	50 gtt/min
9.	33 gtt/min	36.	33 gtt/min
10.	67 gtt/min	37.	65 gtt/min
11.	13 gtt/min	38.	38 gtt/min
12.	33 gtt/min	39.	30 gtt/min
13.	21 gtt/min	40.	50 gtt/min
14.	28 gtt/min	41.	50 gtt/min
15.	63 gtt/min	42.	25 gtt/min
16.	38 gtt/min	43.	23 gtt/min
17.	31 gtt/min	44.	14 gtt/min
18.	56 gtt/min	45.	63 gtt/min
19.	50 gtt/min	46.	31 gtt/min
20.	31 gtt/min	47.	47 gtt/min
21.	33 gtt/min	48.	17 gtt/min
22.	21 gtt/min	49.	25 gtt/min
23.	50 gtt/min	50.	13 gtt/min
24.	25 gtt/min	51.	28 gtt/min
25.	40 gtt/min	52.	17 gtt/min
26.	27 gtt/min	53.	100 gtt/min
27.	19 gtt/min	54.	36 gtt/min

55. 40 gtt/min
56. 25 gtt/min
57. 33 gtt/min
58. 67 gtt/min
59. 44 gtt/min
60. 13 gtt/min
61. 11 gtt/min
62. 40 gtt/min
63. 17 gtt/min
64. 12 gtt/min
65. 31 gtt/min
66. 17 gtt/min
67. 19 gtt/min
68. 35 gtt/min
69. 15 gtt/min
70. 26 gtt/min
71. 22 gtt/min
72. 25 gtt/min
73. 35 gtt/min
74. 60 gtt/min
75. 33 gtt/min
76. 17 gtt/min
77. 25 gtt/min
78. 42 gtt/min

79. 39 gtt/min
80. 33 gtt/min
81. 37 gtt/min
82. 44 gtt/min
83. 50 gtt/min
84. 29 gtt/min
85. 25 gtt/min
86. 50 gtt/min
87. 21 gtt/min
88. 21 gtt/min
89. 31 gtt/min
90. 33 gtt/min
91. 56 gtt/min
92. 75 gtt/min
93. 42 gtt/min
94. 31 gtt/min
95. 50 gtt/min
96. 83 gtt/min
97. 28 gtt/min
98. 21 gtt/min
99. 25 gtt/min
100. 125 gtt/min
101. 17 gtt/min

Calculating Pediatric Dosages Using Body Weight and Body Surface Area

PEDIATRIC DOSAGE CALCULATIONS

NOTE: *Dosages are not safe if they* exceed *the safe dosage range. The dosage can be less than the safe dosage range. Answers should be properly labeled for accuracy.*

1. The physician orders amprenavir 650 mg tid for a child weighing 66 pounds. The safe dosage for this drug is 22.5 mg/kg of body weight up to 3 times a day.

   What is the safe dose for this child?   _____

   Is the ordered dose safe for this child?   _____

2. Cefdinir is ordered for a child weighing 31 pounds. The safe dosage for cefdinir is 7 mg/kg every 12 hours.

   What is the safe dose for this child?   _____

3. The physician orders azithromycin 200 mg 1 time dose for a child weighing 44 pounds. The safe dosage is 10 mg/kg of body weight.

   What is the safe dose for this child?   _____

   Is this a safe dose for this child?   _____

4. The physician orders cefixime oral 100 mg q12h for a child weighing 12 kg. The safe maximum dose for cefixime oral is 4 mg/kg q12h.

   What is the safe dose for this child?   _____

   Is the ordered dose safe?   _____

5. The physician orders azithromycin 100 mg on days 2 through 5 for a child weighing 44 pounds. The safe dose for days 2 through 5 of this drug is 5 mg/kg of body weight.

   What is the safe dose for this child?   _____

6. The physician orders gentamycin 80 mg IV q8h for a child weighing 22 pounds. The safe dosage range is 6–7.5 mg/kg of body weight/24 hours.

   What is the safe dosage range/dose for this child? _____

   Is the ordered dose safe for this child? _____

7. The safe dosage range for acetaminophen is 10–15 mg/kg of body weight q4h.

   What is the maximum safe dose for a child weighing 33 pounds? _____

8. The safe dosage range for ibuprofen is 20–40 mg/kg/day.

   What is the maximum safe daily dose for a child weighing 25 pounds? _____

9. The safe dosage range of gentamycin is 6–7.5 mg/kg/24 hours.

   What is the maximum safe daily dose for a child weighing 33 pounds? _____

10. The physician orders acetaminophen 200 mg q4h po prn for temperature > 38 degrees C. You are caring for a child weighing 27 pounds with a temperature elevation of 38.2 degrees C. The safe dosage range is 10–15 mg/kg/dose.

   What is the maximum safe dose for this child?   _____

   Is the ordered dose safe for this child?   _____

11. Cefotaxime sodium IV is ordered for a child weighing 18 kg. The safe dosage range for this drug is 50–180 mg/kg/day in 6 divided doses.

   What is the safe **range** for an individual dose for this child?   _____

12. The physician orders acetaminophen 240 mg for a child weighing 45 pounds. The safe dosage range is 10–15 mg/kg/dose.

   What is the maximum safe dose for this child?   _____

   Is the ordered dose safe for this child?   _____

13. The safe dosage range for aztreonam for injection is 30 mg/kg/dose, not to exceed 120 mg/kg/day.

    What is the safe individual dose for a child weighing 66 pounds?   _____

14. The safe dosage for cefaclor is 20 mg/kg/day. The physician orders cefaclor 300 mg q8h for a child weighing 40 kg.

    What is the safe dose for this child?   _____

    Is the ordered dose safe?   _____

15. The physician orders cefadroxil monohydrate 350 mg q12 h for a child weighing 88 pounds. The safe dosage is 20 mg/kg/day.

    What is the safe individual dose for this child?   _____

    Is the dose safe for this child?   _____

16. The physician orders cefazolin sodium 250 mg IV q6h for a child weighing 35 pounds. The safe dosage range for cefazolin sodium is 25–50 mg/kg/day in four divided doses.

    What is the safe individual dose range for this child?   _____

    Is the ordered dose safe?   _____

17. Acetaminophen is ordered for a child weighing 14 pounds. The safe dosage range for acetaminophen is 10–15 mg/kg/dose.

    What is the safe **range** for this child?   _____

18. The physician orders ibuprofen 100 mg q6h for a child weighing 22 pounds. The safe dosage range for ibuprofen is 5–10 mg/kg/dose.

    What is the safe **range** for this child?   _____

    Is the ordered dose safe?   _____

19. The physician orders cefpodoxime proxetil for a child weighing 28 kg. The safe dose for this drug is 5 mg/kg/q12h.

    What is the safe dose for this child? _____

20. The physician orders acetaminophen 160 mg for a child weighing 35 pounds. The safe range for acetaminophen is 10–15 mg/kg/dose.

    What is the safe **range** for this child? _____

    Is this a safe dose for this child? _____

21. The physician orders cefprozil 100 mg q12h for a child weighing 34 pounds. The safe dose for this drug is 7.5 mg/kg q12 h.

    What is the safe dose for this child? _____

    Is the ordered dose safe? _____

22. Ibuprofen is ordered for a child weighing 12 kg. The safe dosage range for ibuprofen is 5–10 mg/kg/dose.

    What is the safe dose **range** for this child? _____

23. Acetaminophen is ordered for a child weighing 49 pounds. The safe dosage range for acetaminophen is 10–15 mg/kg/dose.

    What is the safe **range** for this child? _____

24. Ceftazidime IV has been ordered for a neonate weighing 10 pounds. The safe neonate dosage for ceftazidime is 30 mg/kg q12h.

    What is the safe dose for this neonate? _____

25. Acyclovir 200 mg IV q8h has been ordered for a child weighing 42 pounds. The safe dosage range for acyclovir is 10–20 mg/kg q8h.

    What is the safe dosage **range** for this child? _____

    Is the ordered dose safe for this child? _____

26. Amikacin sulfate IV q8h is ordered for a child weighing 75 pounds. The safe dosage range for this drug is 5–7.5 mg/kg q8h.

    What is the safe dosage **range** for this child?   _____

27. Ceftazidime 400 mg IV tid is ordered for an infant weighing 18 pounds. The safe dosage range for ceftazidime is 30–50 mg/kg q8h.

    What is the safe dosage **range** for this child?   _____

    Is the ordered dose safe?   _____

28. The physician orders acetaminophen 260 mg for a child weighing 41 pounds. The safe dosage range for acetaminophen is 10–15 mg/kg/dose.

    What is the safe **range** for this child?   _____

    Is this a safe dose for this child?   _____

29. Aminocaproic acid is ordered for a child weighing 49 kg. The safe dose for this drug is 100 mg/kg.

    What is the safe dose for this child?   _____

30. The physician orders aminophylline 35 mg/hr continuous IV infusion for a 9-month-old infant weighing 20 pounds. The safe dosage range of aminophylline for this age infant is 0.6–0.7 mg/kg/hr.

    What is the safe dosage **range** for this infant?   _____

    Is the ordered dose safe for this infant?   _____

31. Acetaminophen is ordered for a child weighing 51 pounds. The safe dosage range for acetaminophen is 10–15 mg/kg/dose.

    What is the safe **range** for this child?   _____

32. Ampicillin sodium 250 mg IV q6h is ordered for a child weighing 28 pounds. The safe dosage range of ampicillin sodium is 25–50 mg/kg/24 hours.

    What is the safe dosage **range** for an individual dose for this child?   _____

    Is the ordered dose safe?   _____

33. Digoxin is ordered for an infant weighing 9 pounds. The safe dosage range for this drug is 35–60 mcg/kg/dose.

    What is the safe dosage **range** for this infant?   _____

34. Ceftriaxone sodium is ordered for a child weighing 37 pounds. The safe dosage range for this drug is 50–75 mg/kg/day.

    What is the safe daily dosage **range** for this child?   _____

35. Acetaminophen is ordered for a child weighing 23 pounds. The safe dosage range for acetaminophen is 10–15 mg/kg/dose.

    What is the safe **range** for this child?   _____

36. The physician orders cephalexin 250 mg q6h for a child weighing 29 kg. The safe dosage range for cephalexin is 75–100 mg/kg/day in 4 divided doses.

    What is the maximum safe individual dose for this child?   _____

    Is the ordered dose safe for this child?   _____

37. Cephradine is ordered for a child weighing 37 pounds. The safe dosage range of this drug is 75–100 mg/kg/day in 4 divided doses.

    What is the safe dosage **range** for an individual dose for this child? _____

38. Chloral hydrate 500 mg is ordered for conscious sedation for a child weighing 46 pounds. The safe dosage range for chloral hydrate in children is 20–25 mg/kg.

    What is the maximum safe dose for this child? _____

    Is the ordered dose safe for this child? _____

39. Chlorambucil is ordered for a child weighing 30 kg. The safe dosage range for chlorambucil is 0.1–0.2 mg/kg.

    What is the safe dosage **range** for this child? _____

40. Digoxin 100 mcg po is ordered for a child weighing 88 pounds. The safe dosage range of digoxin is 0.008–0.012 mg/kg/dose.

    What is the safe dosage **range** for this child? _____

    Is the ordered dose safe? _____

41. Ibuprofen is ordered for a child weighing 9 kg. The safe dosage range for ibuprofen is 5–10 mg/kg/dose, not to exceed 40 mg/kg/day.

    What is the safe dosage **range** for this child?   _____

42. The physician orders acetaminophen 285 mg for a child weighing 19 kg. The safe dosage range for acetaminophen is 10–15 mg/kg/dose.

    What is the safe dosage **range** for this child?   _____

    Is the ordered dose safe for this child?   _____

43. Ampicillin sodium IV is ordered for a child weighing 34 pounds. The safe dosage range of this drug is 25–50 mg/kg/24 hours.

    What is the safe daily dose for this child?   _____

44. Chlorothiazide 300 mg po bid is ordered for a child weighing 61 pounds. The safe dosage of this drug is 22 mg/kg/day in 2 divided doses.

    What is the safe dosage for this child?   _____

    Is the ordered dose safe?   _____

45. Acetaminophen is ordered for a child weighing 7 kg. The safe dosage range for acetaminophen is 10–15 mg/kg/dose.

    What is the safe dosage **range** for this child?   _____

46. Aminophylline IV is ordered for a 4-year-old child weighing 31 pounds. The safe dosage range of aminophylline for this age child is 0.8–1.2 mg/kg/hr.

    What is the safe dosage **range** for this child?   _____

47. Amikacin sulfate IV 400 mg q12h is ordered for a child weighing 42 kg. The safe dosage range of amikacin sulfate is 15–22.5 mg/kg/day in 2 divided doses.

    What is the safe individual dosage **range** for this child?   _____

    Is the ordered dose safe?   _____

48. Clarithromycin is ordered for a child weighing 12 kilograms. The safe dosage of this drug is 15 mg/kg q12h.

    What is the safe dose of clarithromycin for this child?   _____

49. The physician orders clindamycin 200 mg IV q6h for a child weighing 40 pounds. The safe dosage range of clindamycin is 5–10 mg/kg/dose.

    What is the safe dosage **range** for this child?   _____

    Is the ordered dose safe?   _____

50. Digoxin is ordered for a 2-year-old child weighing 29 pounds. The safe dosage range of digoxin for this age child is 25–35 mcg/kg/daily dose.

    What is the **maximum** daily safe dose for this child?   _____

51. Aminophylline 2 mg/hr IV is ordered for a 5-month-old infant weighing 11 pounds. The safe dosage range of aminophylline for this age infant is 0.5 mg/kg/hr.

    What is the safe hourly dose for this infant?   _____

    Is the ordered dose safe?   _____

52. Clonazepam 300 mcg po q8h is ordered for a child weighing 68 pounds. The safe dosage range for this drug is 0.01–0.03 mg/kg/day in 3 divided doses.

    What is the safe individual dose for this child? _____

    Is the ordered dose safe? _____

53. Cloxacillin sodium 500 mg IV q6h is ordered for a child weighing 19 kg. The safe dose for this drug is 25 mg/kg/dose.

    What is the safe individual dose for this child? _____

    Is the ordered dose safe? _____

54. The physician orders codeine sulfate for a child weighing 23 pounds. The safe dose for this drug is 0.5 mg/kg.

    What is the safe dose for this child? _____

55. The physician orders diazepam 1 mg po q6h for a child weighing 28 pounds. The safe dose for this drug is 0.5 mg/kg/dose.

    What is the safe dose for this child?   _____

    Is the ordered dose safe?   _____

56. The physician orders dolasetron mesylate 35 mg IV prior to chemotherapy for a child weighing 43 pounds. The safe dose for this drug is 1.8 mg/kg/dose.

    What is the safe dose for this child?   _____

    Is the ordered dose safe?   _____

57. Cloxacillin sodium 500 mg IV q6h is ordered for a child weighing 50 pounds. The safe dose of this drug for a child of this weight is 100 mg/kg/day in 4 divided doses.

    What is the safe dose for this child?   _____

    Is the ordered dose safe?   _____

58. The physician orders diazepam for a 10-year-old child weighing 64 pounds. The safe dose of this drug for children this age is 0.3 mg/kg/dose.

    What is the safe individual dose for this child?   _____

59. The physician orders dolasetron 12.5 mg IV for a 5-year-old child weighing 42 pounds. The safe dose of this drug for prevention of postoperative nausea and vomiting is 0.35 mg/kg.

    What is the safe dose for this child?   _____

    Is the ordered dose safe?   _____

60. Doxycycline is ordered for a child weighing 94 pounds. The safe dose of this drug is 2.2 mg/kg per dose.

    What is the safe dose for this child?   _____

61. Etanercept 12.5 mg SC is ordered for a child weighing 89 pounds. The safe dose of this drug is 0.4 mg/kg.

    What is the safe dose for this child? _____

    Is the ordered dose safe for this child? _____

62. Fluconazole is ordered for a child weighing 66 pounds. The safe dose of this drug is 3 mg/kg/day.

    What is the safe daily dose for this child? _____

63. The physician orders furosemide 10 mg po each day for an infant weighing 11 pounds. The safe dosage range for this drug is 1–2 mg/kg/dose.

    What is the safe **maximum** dose for this child? _____

    Is the ordered dose safe? _____

64. Ganciclovir sodium 100 mg IV q12h has been ordered for a child weighing 46 pounds. The safe dosage for this drug is 5 mg/kg/day.

    What is the safe daily dose for this child?   _____

    Is the ordered dose safe?   _____

65. The physician orders glucagon for a child weighing 40 pounds. The safe dose of this drug is 20–30 mcg/kg.

    What is the safe dose for this child?   _____

66. Haloperidol 0.75 mg po q12h is ordered for a child weighing 64 pounds. The safe dosage range for this drug is 50–75 mcg/kg/day.

    What is the safe individual **milligram** dosage range for this child?   _____

    Is the ordered dose safe?   _____

67. Fluconazole 25 mg po tid is ordered for a child weighing 55 pounds. The safe dose of this drug is 3 mg/kg/day.

    What is the safe daily dose for this child? _____

    Is the ordered dose safe? _____

68. The physician orders furosemide 20 mg po for a child weighing 32 pounds. The safe dosage range of this drug is 1–2 mg/kg/dose.

    What is the safe maximum dose for this child _____

    Is the ordered dose safe? _____

69. Ganciclovir sodium 40 mg IV q12h has been ordered for a child weighing 21 kg. The safe dosage range of this drug is 2.5 mg/kg/dose.

    What is the safe dose for this child? _____

    Is the ordered dose safe? _____

70. The physician orders glucagon 0.3 mg IV for an infant weighing 23 pounds. The safe dosage range of this drug is 20–30 mcg/kg.

    What is the safe maximum milligram dose for this child?   _____

    Is the ordered dose safe?   _____

71. Haloperidol 2 mg q12h was ordered for a child weighing 60 pounds. The safe dose of this drug is 50–75 mcg/kg/day.

    What is the safe **milligram** dose for this child?   _____

    Is the ordered dose safe?   _____

72. Lamivudine (3TC) 120 mg bid is ordered for a child weighing 75 pounds. The safe recommended dose of this drug is 4 mg/kg twice a day.

    The safe dose for this child is   _____

    Is the ordered dose safe?   _____

73. Meropenem 500 mg IV q8h is ordered for a child weighing 55 pounds. The safe dose for this drug is 20–40 mg/kg/dose.

    What is the safe **range** for this child?   _____

    Is the ordered dose safe?   _____

74. Minocycline hydrochloride is ordered for a child weighing 30 kg. The safe dose of this drug is 2 mg/kg q12h.

    What is the safe dose for this child?   _____

75. Minoxidil is ordered for a child weighing 31 pounds. The safe dosage range for this drug is 0.25–1.0 mg/kg/day.

    What is the safe dosage **range** for this child?   _____

76. Phenobarbital 40 mg tid is ordered for a child weighing 44 pounds. The safe dosage range for this drug is 3–6 mg/kg/day.

    What is the safe daily dosage **range** for this child?   _____

    Is the ordered dose safe?   _____

77. Phenobarbital is ordered for a child weighing 10 kg. The safe dosage range for this drug is 3–6 mg/kg/day.

    What is the safe dosage **range** for this child?   _____

78. Spectinomycin hydrochloride 2 g IM is ordered for a child weighing 77 pounds. The safe dose for this drug is 40 mg/kg in a 1 time dose.

    What is the safe dose for this child?   _____

    Is the ordered dose safe?   _____

79. Sulfadiazine is ordered for a child weighing 41 pounds. The safe dose of this drug is 75 mg/kg/day in 6 divided doses.

    What is the safe individual dose for this child?   _____

80. Theophylline 75 mg po q6h is ordered for a child weighing 44 pounds. The safe dosage for this drug is 4 mg/kg/dose.

    What is the safe dose for this child?   _____

    Is the ordered dose safe?   _____

81. A child weighing 11 kg is to be started on minoxidil. The initial dose for this agent is 0.2 mg/kg/dose.

    What is the safe dose for this child?   _____

82. Spectinomycin hydrochloride 1.5 g IM is ordered for a child weighing 90 pounds. The safe dose for this drug is 40 mg/kg in a single IM dose.

    What is the safe **gram** dose for this child?   _____

    Is the ordered dose safe?   _____

83. Phenobarbital is ordered for a child weighing 22 kg. The safe dosage range for this drug is 3–6 mg/kg/dose.

    What is the safe **range** for this child?   _____

84. Valproic acid is ordered for an 11-year-old child weighing 60 pounds. The safe dosage range for this drug is 10–15 mg/kg/day for children older than 10 years.

    What is the safe dosage **range** for this child?   _____

85. Vecuronium bromide 5 mg is ordered IV for induction of anesthesia in a child weighing 110 pounds. The safe dose of this drug is 0.08–0.1 mg/kg.

    What is the safe dosage **range** for this child?   _____

    Is the ordered dose safe for this child?   _____

86. Vancomycin hydrochloride 300 mg IV q8h is ordered for a child weighing 48 pounds. The safe dosage for this drug is 10 mg/kg/dose.

    What is the safe dose for this child?   _____

    Is the ordered dose safe?   _____

87. Oxcarbazepine is being ordered for a child weighing 53 pounds. The safe dosage range for this drug is 8–10 mg/kg/dose, not to exceed 600 mg/day.

    What is the safe individual dosage **range** for this child?   _____

88. Atropine sulfate 1/150 gr IV is ordered for a child weighing 13 kg. The safe dosage range for this drug is 0.01–0.03 mg/kg/dose.

    What is the safe dosage **range** for this child? _____

    Is the ordered dose safe? _____

89. Azathioprine sodium 40 mg IV qd is ordered for a child weighing 22 pounds. The safe dosage range for this drug is 3–5 mg/kg/24 hours.

    What is the safe dosage **range** for this child? _____

    Is the ordered dose safe? _____

90. Aztreonam 1 g IV q8h is ordered for a 60-pound child with cystic fibrosis. The safe dose for this drug used to treat infections in children with cystic fibrosis is 50 mg/kg q8h.

    What is the safe **gram** dose for this child? _____

    Is the ordered dose safe? _____

91. Aztreonam 500 mg IV q6h is ordered for a child weighing 56 pounds. The safe dose for this drug is 30 mg/kg q6h.

    What is the safe dose for this child?   _____

    Is the ordered dose safe?   _____

92. Buprenorphine hydrochloride 0.3 mg IV is ordered for a child weighing 50 kg. The safe range of this drug is 2–6 mcg kg/dose.

    What is the safe dosage **range** for this child?   _____

    Is the ordered dose safe?   _____

93. Zidovudine IV 12 mg/hr is ordered to infuse a child weighing 12 kg. The safe range for this drug is 0.5–1.8 mg/kg/hr.

    What is the safe dosage **rate** for this child?   _____

    Is the ordered dose safe?   _____

94. Verapamil hydrochloride IV is ordered for a child weighing 24 pounds. The safe individual dosage range of this drug is 0.1–0.3 mg/kg.

    What is the safe dosage **range** for this child?   _____

95. Vancomycin hydrochloride is ordered for a child weighing 34 kg. The safe dose for this drug is 10 mg/kg/dose.

    What is the safe dose for this child?   _____

96. Tobramycin sulfate IV 50 mg q8h is ordered for a child weighing 47 pounds. The safe dosage range for this drug is 6–7.5 mg/kg/24 hours in 3 divided doses.

    What is the safe individual dose range for this child?   _____

    Is the ordered dose safe?   _____

97. Tacrolimus is ordered for a child weighing 18 kg who had a liver transplant 12 hours ago. The safe dose for this drug is 0.03–0.05 mg/kg/day in 2 divided doses.

    What is the safe individual dose **range** for this child?   _____

98. Ranitidine 10 mg IV is ordered for a child weighing 28 pounds. The safe dosage range for this drug is 2–4 mg/kg/day in equally divided doses every 8 hours.

    What is the safe individual dosage **range** for this child?   _____

    Is the ordered dose safe?   _____

99. Propranolol hydrochloride 0.5 mg IV is ordered for a child weighing 11 pounds. The safe dosage range for this agent is 10–100 mcg/kg/dose.

    What is the safe milligram dosage **range** for this child?   _____

    Is the ordered dose safe?   _____

100. Procainamide hydrochloride IV is ordered for a child weighing 10 kg. The safe dosage range for this drug is 2–5 mg/kg/dose.

    What is the safe dosage **range** for this child?   _____

Answers for Unit VIII

1. 675 mg/dose
   Yes, dose safe
2. 98.6 mg/dose
3. 200 mg/dose
   Yes, dose safe
4. 48 mg/dose
   No, dose not safe
5. 100 mg/day
6. 20–25 mg/dose
   No, dose not safe
7. 225 mg/dose
8. 454.5 mg/24 hours
9. 112.5 mg/24 hours
10. 184 mg/dose
    No, dose not safe
11. 150–540 mg/dose
12. 306.8 mg/dose
    Yes, dose safe
13. 900 mg/dose
14. 267 mg/dose
    No, dose not safe
15. 400 mg/dose
    Yes, dose safe
16. 99.4–198.9 mg/dose
    No, dose not safe
17. 63.6–95.5 mg/dose

18. 50–100 mg/dose
    Yes, dose safe
19. 140 mg q12h
20. 159–238.6 mg/dose
    Yes, dose safe
21. 115.9 mg/dose
    Yes, dose safe
22. 60–120 mg/dose
23. 222.7–334.1 mg/dose
24. 136.4 mg q12h
25. 190.9–381.8 mg/q8h
    Yes, dose safe
26. 170.5–255.7 mg/q8h
27. 245.5–409.1 mg/q8h
    Yes, dose safe
28. 186.4–279.5 mg/dose
    Yes, dose safe
29. 4900 mg/dose or 4.9 g/dose
30. 5.5–6.4 mg/dose
    No, dose not safe
31. 231.8–347.7 mg/dose
32. 79.5–159 mg/dose
    No, dose not safe
33. 143–245.5 mcg/dose
34. 840.9–1261.4 mg/day
35. 104.5–156.8 mg/dose

36. 725 mg/dose
    Yes, dose safe
37. 315.3–420.5 mg/dose
38. 522.7 mg/dose
    Yes, dose safe
39. 3–6 mg/dose
40. 320–480 mcg/dose
    Yes, dose safe, but low
41. 45–90 mg/dose, not to exceed 360 mg/day
42. 190–285 mg/dose
    Yes, dose safe
43. 386.4–772.7 mg/day
44. 305 mg/dose
    Yes, dose safe
45. 70–105 mg/dose
46. 11.3–16.9 mg/hr
47. 315–472.5 mg/dose
    Yes, dose safe
48. 180 mg/dose q12h
49. 90.9–181.8 mg/dose
    No, dose not safe
50. 461.4 mcg/daily dose
51. 2.5 mg/hr
    Yes, dose safe
52. 0.1–0.3 mg or 100–300 mcg/dose
    Yes, dose safe
53. 475 mg/dose
    No, dose not safe

54. 5.2 mg/dose
55. 6.4 mg/dose
    Yes, dose safe
56. 35.2 mg/dose
    Yes, dose safe
57. 568.2 mg/dose
    Yes, dose safe
58. 8.7 mg/dose
59. 6.7 mg/dose
    No, dose not safe
60. 94 mg/dose
61. 16.2 mg/dose
    Yes, dose safe
62. 90 mg/day
63. 10 mg/dose
    Yes, dose safe
64. 104.5 mg/day
    No, dose not safe
65. 363.6–545.5 mcg/dose
66. 0.73–1.1 mg/dose
    Yes, dose safe
67. 75 mg/dose
    Yes, dose safe
68. 29.1 mg/dose
    Yes, dose safe
69. 52.5 mg/dose
    Yes, dose safe
70. 0.3 mg/dose
    Yes, dose safe

71. 0.7–1.0 mg/dose
No, dose not safe

72. 136.4 mg/dose
Yes, dose safe

73. 500–1000 mg/dose
Yes, dose safe

74. 60 mg q12h

75. 3.5–14.1 mg/day

76. 60–120 mg/day
Yes, dose safe

77. 30–60 mg/day

78. 1.4 g/dose
No, dose not safe

79. 233 mg/dose

80. 80 mg/dose
Yes, dose safe

81. 2.2 mg/dose

82. 1.6 g/dose
Yes, dose safe

83. 66–132 mg/dose

84. 272.7–409.1 mg/day

85. 4–5 mg/dose
Yes, dose safe

86. 218.2 mg/dose
No, dose not safe

87. 192.7–240.9 mg/dose

88. 0.13–0.4 mg/dose; 1/150 gr = 0.4 mg
Yes, dose safe

89. 30–50 mg/day
Yes, dose safe

90. 1.4 g/dose
Yes, dose safe

91. 763.6 mg/q6h
Yes, dose safe

92. 0.1–0.3 mg/dose
Yes, dose safe

93. 6-21.6 mg/hr
Yes, dose safe

94. 1.1–3.3 mg/dose

95. 340 mg/dose

96. 42.7–53.4 mg/dose
Yes, dose safe

97. 0.27–0.45 mg/dose

98. 8.5–17 mg/dose
Yes, dose safe

99. 0.05–0.5 mg/dose
Yes, dose safe

100. 20–50 mg/dose

Advanced Calculations

Answer the following calculation questions.

a. Calculating Infusion Time for IV Fluids and Enteral Feedings

1. 1000 ml bag of 5% dextrose in water with 20 mEq of potassium chloride is to infuse at 125 ml/hr. How long will this bag last? _____

2. 750 ml bag of 0.9% sodium chloride is to infuse at 100 ml/hr. How long will this bag last? _____

3. 720 ml of total parenteral nutrition is programmed into the intravenous infusion pump to infuse at 36 ml/hr. How long will this infusion last? _____

4. 320 ml of packed red blood cells is to infuse at 100 ml/hr. How long will this infusion last? _____

5. 80 ml of 0.45% normal saline is to infuse at 20 drops/minute using microdrip tubing. The drip factor is 60 gtt/ml. How long will this infusion last?   _____

6. 50 ml of cefoxitin 1 gram is to infuse at 67 gtt/min using macrodrip tubing with a drip factor of 20 gtt/ml. How long will this infusion last?   _____

7. 100 ml of gentamycin 80 mg is to infuse at 50 gtt/min using a macrodrip tubing with a drip factor of 15 gtt/min. How long will this infusion last?   _____

8. 25 ml of ondansetron 4 mg is to infuse at 17 gtt/min using a macrodrip tubing with a drip factor of 10 gtt/ml. How long will this infusion last?   _____

9. The physician orders clindamycin 900 mg in 100 ml of 0.9% normal saline to infuse at 10 mg/min. How long will this infusion last?   _____

10. The physician orders aminophylline 500 mg in 1 L of 5% dextrose in water to infuse at 25 mg/hr. How long will this infusion last?   _____

11. The physician orders 500 ml bolus of 0.9 sodium chloride to infuse at 200 ml/hr. How long will this infusion last?   _____

12. The physician orders oxicillin sodium 500 mg in 50 ml of 5% dextrose/0.9% normal saline to infuse at 100 ml/hr. How long will this infusion last?   _____

13. The physician orders rifampin 600 mg to infuse at 200 mg/hr. The pharmacy sends you 600 mg rifampin in 500 milliliters 5% dextrose in water. How long will this infusion last?   _____

14. The physician orders vancomycin 750 mg to infuse at 7.5 mg/kg/hr for a client weighing 50 kg. The pharmacy sends vancomycin 750 mg in 250 ml 0.9% normal saline. How long will this infusion last?   _____

15. The physician orders vancomycin 450 mg to infuse at 7.5 mg/kg/hr for a client weighing 132 pounds. The pharmacy sends vancomycin 450 mg in 100 ml of 5% dextrose in water. How long will this infusion last?

_____

16. 500 ml of 0.9% normal saline is to infuse at 150 ml/ hour. How long will this infusion last?

_____

17. 1000 ml of 5% dextrose/½ normal saline with 20 mEq of potassium chloride is to infuse at 100 ml/hr. How long will this infusion last?

_____

18. 1000 ml of 0.9% normal saline is to infuse at 75 ml/hr. How long will this infusion last?

_____

19. 1000 ml of 5% dextrose in water is to infuse at 50 ml/hr. How long will this infusion last?

_____

20. 1000 ml of 5% dextrose/0.9% normal saline is to infuse at 80 ml/hr. How long will this infusion last?   _____

21. 180 ml of 20% intralipids is programmed to infuse at 10 ml/hr. How long will this infusion last?   _____

22. The physician orders aminophylline continuous infusion at 20 mg/hr. The pharmacy sends 400 mg of aminophylline in 1 L of 5% dextrose in water. How long will this infusion last?   _____

23. 320 ml of packed red blood cells are ordered to infuse at 40 ml/hr for the first 30 minutes and 100 ml/hr after the first 30 minutes. How long will this infusion last?   _____

24. The physician orders ½ unit of packed red blood cells to infuse at 50 ml/hr. The blood bank provides 160 ml of packed red blood cells. How long will this infusion last?   _____

25. The physician orders clindamycin 300 mg in 100 ml 0.9% normal saline to infuse at 10 mg/min. How long will this infusion last?   _____

26. The physician orders cytarabine 6 mg/kg/day for a client weighing 154 pounds. The pharmacy sends 420 mg cytarabine in 1000 ml of 0.9% normal saline. How long will this infusion last?   _____

27. 500 ml of 5% dextrose/½ normal saline is to infuse at 30 ml/hr. How long will this infusion last?   _____

28. 1060 ml of total parenteral nutrition is programmed to infuse at 53 ml/hr. How long will this infusion last?   _____

29. 1000 ml of total parenteral nutrition is programmed to infuse at 60 ml/hr. How long will this infusion last?   _____

30. 600 ml of IV solution is in the IV bag when you start your shift at 0700.   _____
    The infusion rate is 100 ml/hr. At what time will this infusion be com-
    pleted?

31. 350 ml of IV solution is in the IV bag when you start your shift at 1900.   _____
    The infusion rate is 125 ml/hr. At what time will this infusion be com-
    pleted?

32. 950 ml of IV solution is in the IV bag when you start your shift at 1500.   _____
    The infusion rate is 100 ml/hr. At what time will this infusion be com-
    pleted?

33. 700 ml of IV solution is in the IV bag when you start your shift at 2300.   _____
    The infusion rate is 80 ml/hr. At what time will this infusion be com-
    pleted?

34. 400 ml of IV solution is in the IV bag when you start your shift at 0600.   _____
    The infusion rate is 75 ml/hr. At what time will this infusion be com-
    pleted?

35. 300 ml of IV solution is in the IV bag when you start your shift at 0700. The infusion rate is 50 ml/hr. At what time will this infusion be completed?

_____

36. 200 ml of IV solution is in the IV bag when you start your shift at 1900. The infusion rate is 40 ml/hr. At what time will this infusion be completed?

_____

37. 400 ml of IV solution is in the IV bag when you start your shift at 2300. The infusion rate is 25 ml/hr. At what time will this infusion be completed?

_____

38. 50 ml of IV solution is in the IV bag when you start your shift at 0700. The infusion rate is 200 ml/hr. At what time will this infusion be completed?

_____

39. 100 ml of IV solution is in the IV bag when you start your shift at 1500. The infusion rate is 10 ml/hr. At what time will this infusion be completed?

_____

40. Total parenteral nutrition is to infuse at 36 ml/hr. When you start your shift at 1100 the IV infusion pump reads that 750 ml remain in the IV bag. At what time will the infusion be completed?

41. Intralipids 20% are infusing at 8 ml/hr. When you start your shift at 0700 the IV infusion pump reads that 72 ml remain in the IV infusion. At what time will the infusion be completed?

42. The physician orders continuous ½ strength enteral feedings to infuse at 60 ml/hr. How much water will you need to add to one 8 ounce can to make this concentration?

    How long will this infusion last?

43. The physician orders continuous ¼ strength enteral feedings to infuse at 20 ml/hr. How much water will you need to add to 50 ml of feeding to make this concentration?

    How long will this infusion last?

44. The client has 500 ml of enteral feedings infusing at 75 ml/hr when you begin your shift. How long will this enteral feeding last?   _____

45. The order for enteral feedings reads to use one 8-ounce can of enteral feeding and infuse at 40 ml/hr. How long will this enteral feeding last?   _____

46. The physician orders enteral feedings to infuse at 80 ml/hr. The feeding bag contains 680 ml when you begin your shift at 0700. At what time will the infusion be completed?   _____

47. The physician orders enteral feedings to infuse at 35 ml/hr. The feeding bag contains 350 ml when you begin your shift at 2300. At what time will the infusion be completed?   _____

48. When you begin your shift at 0800, the client's enteral feeding bag contains 480 ml. The rate of the feeding is 30 ml/hr. At what time will the infusion be completed?   _____

49. When you begin your shift at 1500, the client's enteral feeding bag   _____
contains 240 ml. The rate of the feeding is 15 ml/hr. How long will the
infusion last?

50. When you begin your shift at 0700, the client's enteral feeding bag   _____
contains 240 ml. The physician's order reads to start enteral feedings
at 30 ml/hr and q2h increase the feeding by 10 ml until a goal of 80
ml/hr. At what time will this feeding be completed?

b. Intravenous Drug Concentrations

1. The physician orders regular insulin to infuse intravenously at 10   _____
   units/hour. The pharmacy sends 500 units of regular insulin in 100 ml
   of 0.9% normal saline. The intravenous infusion pump should be programmed to infuse how many milliliters/hour to deliver the ordered
   dose?

2. The physician orders heparin sodium to infuse intravenously at 1100   _____
   units/hr. The pharmacy sends 25,000 units of heparin in 500 ml of ½
   normal saline solution. The intravenous infusion pump should be programmed to infuse how many milliliters/hour to deliver the ordered
   dose?

3. The physician orders heparin sodium to infuse intravenously at 750 units/hr. The pharmacy sends 20,000 units of heparin in 500 ml of 0.9% normal saline solution. The intravenous infusion pump should be programmed to infuse how many ml/hour to deliver the ordered dose?

_____

4. The physician orders potassium chloride to infuse at 10 mEq/hour. The pharmacy sends 50 mEq of potassium chloride in 250 ml of 5% dextrose in water. The intravenous infusion pump should be programmed to infuse how many ml/hr to deliver the ordered dose?

_____

5. Aminophylline 500 mg in 1000 ml of 5% dextrose in water to infuse at 25 mg/hr. The intravenous infusion pump should be programmed to infuse how many ml/hr to deliver the ordered dose?

_____

6. The physician orders regular insulin 5 units per hour intravenous to be administered at a rate of 25 ml/hr. Available is 500 ml of 0.9% normal saline and a vial of regular insulin. How many units of insulin would you add to the IV solution to deliver the ordered rate?

_____

7. The physician orders heparin sodium 800 units/hr intravenously. The pharmacy sends 20,000 U heparin sodium in 500 ml of 5% dextrose in water. How many ml/hr should be infused to deliver the ordered rate?

_____

8. Corticotropin 15 units in 500 ml of 5% dextrose in water is to be
   infused at 0.06 units/min. How many units/hr should be infused to
   deliver the ordered rate?

   The intravenous infusion pump should be programmed to deliver how
   many ml/hr?

9. The physician orders isoproterenol hydrochloride to be infused intravenously at 5 mcg/min. The pharmacy sends 2 mg isoproterenol hydrochloride in 500 ml of 5% dextrose in water. The intravenous
   infusion pump should be programmed to deliver how many ml/hr?

10. The physician orders lidocaine hydrochloride to infuse at 2 mg/min.
    The pharmacy sends 1 gram lidocaine hydrochloride in 250 ml of 5%
    dextrose in water. The intravenous infusion pump should be pro-
    grammed to deliver how many ml/hr?

11. The physician orders morphine sulfate to infuse intravenously at 3
    mg/hr. The pharmacy sends 60 mg morphine sulfate in 250 ml of ½
    normal saline. The intravenous infusion pump should be programmed
    to deliver how many ml/hr?

12. The physician orders nitroglycerin to infuse intravenously at 600 mcg/hr. The pharmacy sends 10 mg nitroglycerin in 250 ml of 5% dextrose in water. The intravenous infusion pump should be programmed to deliver how many ml/hr?

      _____

13. The physician orders procainamide hydrochloride to infuse intravenously at 5 mg/min. The pharmacy sends 1 gram procainamide hydrochloride in 500 ml of 5% dextrose in water. The intravenous infusion pump should be programmed to deliver how many ml/hr?

      _____

14. The physician orders nitroprusside sodium to infuse intravenously at 0.1 mg/min. The pharmacy sends 50 mg nitroprusside sodium in 500 ml of 5% dextrose in water. The intravenous infusion pump should be programmed to deliver how many ml/hr?

      _____

15. The physician orders norepinephrine to infuse intravenously at 10 mcg/min. The pharmacy sends 4 mg norepinephrine in 500 ml of 5% dextrose in water. The intravenous infusion pump should be programmed to deliver how many ml/hr?

      _____

16. The physician orders dopamine hydrochloride to infuse intravenously at 2 mg/hr. The pharmacy sends 200 mg dopamine hydrochloride in 250 ml of IV fluids. The intravenous infusion pump should be programmed to deliver how many ml/hr?

      _____

17. The physician orders regular insulin to infuse at 5 units/hr. The pharmacy sends 100 units regular insulin in 250 ml of 0.9% normal saline. The intravenous infusion pump should be programmed to deliver how many ml/hr?

     _____

18. The physician orders regular insulin to infuse at 7 units/hr. The pharmacy sends 100 units regular insulin in 100 ml of 0.9% normal saline. The intravenous infusion pump should be programmed to deliver how many ml/hr?

     _____

19. The physician orders regular insulin to infuse at 9 units/hr. The pharmacy sends 100 units regular insulin in 240 ml of 0.9% normal saline. The intravenous infusion pump should be programmed to deliver how many ml/hr?

     _____

20. The physician orders aminophylline to infuse intravenously at 35 mg/hr. Aminophylline 500 mg in 1000 ml of 5% dextrose in water is sent from the pharmacy. The intravenous infusion pump should be programmed to deliver how many ml/hr?

     _____

21. The physician orders dobutamine to infuse intravenously at 300 mcg/min. The pharmacy sends 250 mg dobutamine in 250 ml of 5% dextrose in water. The intravenous infusion pump should be programmed to deliver how many ml/hr?

     _____

22. The physician orders nitroglycerin to infuse at 10 mcg/min. The pharmacy sends 50 mg nitroglycerin in 250 ml of 5% dextrose in water. The intravenous infusion pump should be programmed to deliver how many ml/hr?

_____

23. The physician orders norepinephrine to infuse at 12 mcg/min. The pharmacy sends 4 mg norepinephrine in 250 ml of 5% dextrose in water. The intravenous infusion pump should be programmed to deliver how many ml/hr?

_____

24. The physician orders diltiazem hydrochloride to infuse IV at 10 mg/hr. The pharmacy sends 125 mg diltiazem hydrochloride in 250 ml of 0.9% normal saline. The intravenous infusion pump should be programmed to deliver how many ml/hr?

_____

25. The physician orders aminophylline to infuse at 30 mg/hr. The pharmacy sends 250 mg aminophylline in 500 ml of 5% dextrose in water. The intravenous infusion pump should be programmed to deliver how many ml/hr?

_____

26. The physician orders heparin to infuse at 1200 units/hr. The pharmacy sends 40,000 units heparin in 500 ml of 5% dextrose in water. The intravenous infusion pump should be programmed to deliver how many ml/hr?

_____

27. The physician orders heparin to infuse at 900 units/hr. The pharmacy sends 25,000 units heparin in 500 ml of 5% dextrose in water. The intravenous infusion pump should be programmed to deliver how many ml/hr?

         _____

28. The physician orders heparin to infuse at 500 units/hr. The pharmacy sends 10,000 units heparin in 250 ml of ½ normal saline. The intravenous infusion pump should be programmed to deliver how many ml/hr?

         _____

29. The physician orders heparin to infuse at 1000 units/hour. The pharmacy sends 25,000 units heparin in 1000 ml of ½ normal saline. The intravenous infusion pump should be programmed to deliver how many ml/hr?

         _____

30. The physician orders regular insulin to infuse at 11 units/hr. The pharmacy sends 500 units regular insulin in 500 ml of 0.9% normal saline. The intravenous infusion pump should be programmed to deliver how many ml/hr?

         _____

31. The physician orders regular insulin to infuse at 4 units/hr. The pharmacy sends 250 units regular insulin in 250 ml of 0.9% normal saline. The intravenous infusion pump should be programmed to deliver how many ml/hr?

         _____

32. The physician orders regular insulin 5 units/hr to be administered intravenously at a rate of 30 ml/hr. Available is 250 ml of 0.9% normal saline and a vial of regular insulin. How many units of the insulin would you add to the IV solution to deliver the ordered rate?

_____

33. The physician orders regular insulin 12 units/hr to be administered intravenously at a rate of 25 ml/hr. Available is 500 ml of 0.9% normal saline and a vial of regular insulin. How many units of the insulin would you add to the IV solution to deliver the ordered rate?

_____

34. The physician orders potassium chloride to infuse at 10 mEq/hr. The pharmacy sends you 100 ml of 5% dextrose in water containing 20 mEq of potassium chloride. The intravenous infusion pump should be programmed to administer how many ml/hr?

_____

35. The physician orders potassium chloride to infuse at 20 mEq/hr. The pharmacy sends you 100 ml of 5% dextrose in water containing 20 mEq of potassium chloride. The intravenous infusion pump should be programmed to administer how many ml/hr?

_____

36. The physician orders potassium chloride to infuse at 2 mEq/hr. The pharmacy sends you 1 liter of 5% dextrose/½ normal saline with 40 mEq. The intravenous infusion pump should be programmed to deliver how many ml/hr?

_____

37. The physician orders magnesium sulfate 2 grams/hr. The pharmacy provides you with 1000 ml Ringer's lactate with 50 grams of magnesium sulfate. The intravenous infusion pump should be programmed to administer how many ml/hr?

_____

38. The physician orders oxytocin 2 units/hr. The pharmacy provides you with 20 units oxytocin in 1000 ml of lactated Ringer's. The intravenous infusion pump should be programmed to administer how many ml/hr?

_____

39. The physician orders dopamine 1.5 mg/hr. The pharmacy sends 800 mg dopamine in 1 L of 0.9% normal saline. The intravenous infusion pump should be programmed to administer how many ml/hr?

_____

40. The physician orders isoproterenol to infuse at 5 mcg/min. The pharmacy sends 2 mg isoproterenol in 500 ml 5% dextrose in water. The intravenous infusion pump should be programmed to administer how many ml/hr?

_____

41. The physician orders oxytoxcin 4 units/hr. The pharmacy sends 60 units oxytocin in 1000 ml of lactated Ringer's. The intravenous infusion pump should be programmed to administer how many ml/hr?

_____

42. The physician orders heparin 10,000 units in 500 ml of 5% dextrose   _____
    in water to infuse at 1200 units/hr. The vial of heparin sent from the
    pharmacy is 5000 units/ml. How many milliliters of heparin should you
    add to the IV solution?

43. The physician orders 1 gram ampicillin in 50 ml of 0.9% normal saline.   _____
    The pharmacy sends you a vial of ampicillin powder to be reconsti-
    tuted in 2 ml of sterile water for a concentration of 500 mg/ml. How
    many milliliters should you add to the IV solution?

44. The physician orders penicillin oral solution 100,000 units q6h. The   _____
    pharmacy sends you 125 mg (200,000 units) penicillin per 5 ml. How
    many milliliters will you administer to deliver the ordered dose?

45. The physician orders aminophylline 150 mg IV q6h. The pharmacy   _____
    sends a 250 mg/10 ml solution of aminophylline. How much amino-
    phylline will you add to 50 ml of 5% dextrose in water to administer
    the ordered dose in 30 minutes?

46. The physician orders aminophylline 50 mg/hr for a 10-year-old child.   _____
    The pharmacy sends 250 mg aminophylline in 250 ml of 5% dextrose
    in water. The infusion pump should be programmed to administer
    how many ml/hr?

47. The physician orders potassium chloride to infuse at 10 mEq/hr. The pharmacy sends you 50 mEq potassium chloride in 100 ml of 0.9% normal saline. The intravenous infusion pump should be programmed at how many ml/hr?

    _____

48. The physician orders ondansetron to infuse 1 mg/hr over 24 hours. The pharmacy sends you 25 mg of ondansetron in 1000 ml of 0.9% normal saline. The intravenous infusion pump should be programmed at how many ml/hr?

    _____

49. The physician orders sodium bicarbonate to infuse at 10 mEq/hr. The pharmacy sends you 250 mEq sodium bicarbonate in 1 L of 5% dextrose in water. The intravenous infusion pump should be programmed at how many ml/hr?

    _____

50. The physician orders rifampin 100 mg/hr. The pharmacy sends you 600 mg rifampin in 500 milliliters 5% dextrose in water. The intravenous infusion pump should be programmed at how many ml/hr?

    _____

Answers for Unit IX

a. Calculating Infusion Time for IV Fluids and Enteral Feedings

1. 8 hours
2. 7.5 hours or 7 hours and 30 minutes
3. 20 hours
4. 3 hours and 12 minutes
5. 4 hours
6. 15 minutes
7. 30 minutes
8. 15 minutes
9. 1.5 hours or 1 hour and 30 minutes
10. 20 hours
11. 2.5 hours or 2 hours and 30 minutes
12. 30 minutes
13. 3 hours
14. 2 hours
15. 1 hour
16. 3 hours and 20 minutes
17. 10 hours
18. 13 hours and 20 minutes
19. 20 hours
20. 12.5 hours or 12 hours and 30 minutes
21. 18 hours
22. 20 hours
23. 3 hours and 30 minutes
24. 3 hours and 12 minutes
25. 30 minutes
26. 24 hours

27. 16 hours and 40 minutes
28. 20 hours
29. 16 hours and 40 minutes
30. 1300 or 1:00 pm
31. 2148 or 9:48 pm
32. 0030 or 12:30 am
33. 0745 or 7:45 am
34. 1120 or 11:20 am
35. 1300 or 1:00 pm
36. 2400 or 12:00 am
37. 1500 or 3:00 pm
38. 0715 or 7:15 am
39. 0100 or 1:00 am
40. 0750 or 7:50 am
41. 1600 or 4:00 pm
42. 240 ml H_2O;
    8 hours
43. 150 ml H_2O;
    10 hours
44. 6 hours and 40 minutes
45. 6 hours
46. 1530 or 3:30 pm
47. 0900 or 9:00 am
48. 2400 or 12:00 am
49. 16 hours
50. 1300 or 1:00 pm

b. Intravenous Drug Concentrations

1.	2 ml/hr	26.	15 ml/hr
2.	22 ml/hr	27.	18 ml/hr
3.	18.75 ml/hr	28.	12.5 ml/hr
4.	50 ml/hr	29.	40 ml/hr
5.	50 ml/hr	30.	11 ml/hr
6.	100 units	31.	4 ml/hr
7.	20 ml/hr	32.	42 units
8.	3.6 units/hr; 120 ml/hr	33.	240 units
9.	75 ml/hr	34.	50 ml/hr
10.	30 ml/hr	35.	100 ml/hr
11.	12.5 ml/hr	36.	50 ml/hr
12.	15 ml/hr	37.	40 ml/hr
13.	150 ml/hr	38.	100 ml/hr
14.	60 ml/hr	39.	1.9 ml/hr
15.	75 ml/hr	40.	75 ml/hr
16.	2.5 ml/hr	41.	66.7 ml/hr
17.	12.5 ml/hr	42.	2 ml
18.	7 ml/hr	43.	2 ml
19.	21.6 ml/hr	44.	2.5 ml
20.	70 ml/hr	45.	6 ml
21.	18 ml/hr	46.	50 ml/hr
22.	3 ml/hr	47.	20 ml/hr
23.	45 ml/hr	48.	40 ml/hr
24.	20 ml/hr	49.	40 ml/hr
25.	60 ml/hr	50.	83.3 ml/hr

Comprehensive Examination

1. The physician prescribes phenytoin 200 mg po each day. On hand are capsules labeled 0.1 grams of phenytoin. The nurse should administer _____ capsule(s) per dose.

2. The physician prescribes 600 mg of acyclovir po q4h. On hand are tablets labeled acyclovir 200 mg. The nurse should administer _____ tablet(s) per dose.

3. The physician orders diltiazem hydrochloride gr 1½ po bid. On hand are capsules diltiazem HCl SR 90 mg per capsules. The nurse should administer _____ capsule(s) per dose.

4. The physician orders nitroglycerin 0.3 mg sublingual at the onset of chest pain. May repeat dose in 5 minutes. On hand are nitroglycerin tablet(s) 1/200 gr. The nurse should administer _____ tablet(s) per dose.

5. The physician orders amoxicillin/potassium clavulanate 20 mg/kg/day in 4 divided doses by mouth to a child weighing 44 pounds. The pharmacy sends 100 mg tablets amoxicillin/potassium clavulanate. The nurse should administer _____ tablet(s) per dose to this child.

6. The physician orders acetaminophen 650 mg q4h as needed for pain. The nurse has 325 mg acetaminophen tablets available. The nurse should administer _____ tablet(s) per dose.

7. The physician orders digoxin 0.25 mg po qAM. The nurse has on hand 250 mcg digoxin tablets. The nurse should administer _____ tablet(s) every morning after counting the client's apical pulse.

8. The physician orders 0.15 mg of levothroid to be administered by mouth each morning. The pharmacy sends 150 mcg levothroid tablets. The nurse should administer _____ tablet(s) for each dose.

9. The physician orders oxycodone/APAP 5/325 two tablets every 4 hours as needed for pain. The nurse can administer a maximum of _____ tablets in a 24 hour period.

10. The physician writes an order for acetaminophen 200 mg po for an elderly adult. You have on hand acetaminophen oral liquid 80 mg in 0.8 ml. The nurse should administer _____ ml.

11. The physician orders 180 mg acyclovir po. The pharmacy supplies acyclovir suspension 200 mg/5 ml. The nurse should administer _____ ml.

12. The physician orders amoxicillin/potassium clavulanate 75 mg po q12h. The pharmacy fills the client's prescription with amoxicillin/potassium clavulanate 125 mg/5 ml suspension. The client's parent should be instructed to administer _____ ml.

13. The physician orders acetaminophen 160 mg po for a child. You have on hand acetaminophen 80 mg per 2.5 ml in oral liquid. The nurse should administer _____ ml.

14. The physician orders cefaclor 2 g via gastric tube in 2 divided doses. The pharmacy sends cefaclor 375 mg/5 ml suspension. The nurse should administer _____ ml per dose.

15. The physician orders digoxin elixir 125 mcg po each day. The pharmacy sends digoxin 0.05 mg/ml. The nurse should administer _____ ml per dose after monitoring the client's apical pulse.

16. The physician orders cephalexin HCl 4 g in 4 divided doses po each day for 5 days. The pharmacy supplies cephalexin HCl suspension 250 mg/5 ml. The nurse should instruct the client to take _____ ml per dose.

17. The physician orders clonazepam 5 mg tid po for a client with severe Parkinson's disease. The pharmacy supplies 2 mg tablets. Because the client cannot swallow tablets, the nurse crushes each tablet in 3 ml of water making a concentration of 2 mg/3 ml. The client should receive _____ ml per dose of this solution to receive the ordered dose.

18. The physician orders codeine sulfate ½ gr po. The pharmacy supplies the controlled substances with codeine sulfate oral solution 15 mg/5 ml. The nurse should administer _____ ml per dose.

19. The physician orders haloperidol 3 mg po at hs. The pharmacy fills the prescription with haloperidol oral concentrate 2 mg/ml. The client should be instructed to take _____ ml at bedtime.

20. The physician orders 15 units of Regular insulin and 29 units of NPH insulin SC at 1700 hours. What is the total number units of insulin the nurse will draw up in the syringe and administer? _____

21. The physician orders atropine 1/150 gr SC. The atropine vial is labeled 0.4 mg/ml. The nurse should administer _____ ml SC.

22. The physician orders 525 IU of antihemophilic factor (Factor VIII) IV qd. The pharmacy supplies a the antihemophilic factor in a concentration of 75 IU/5 ml. The nurse should administer _____ ml IV bolus.

23. The physician orders 2500 U heparin sodium SC bid. The pharmacy sends heparin sodium 10,000 U/ml. The nurse should administer _____ ml SC.

24. The physician orders promethazine sulfate 25 mg IV. The label on the vial containing the promethazine sulfate states 25 mg/ml. The IV drug resource states that each 12.5 mg of promethazine sulfate should be diluted with 5 ml of normal saline for injection prior to administration. The nurse should administer a total fluid and medication bolus of _____ ml.

25. The physician orders enoxaparin sodium 30 mg SC bid. The pharmacy sends enoxaparin sodium 60 mg/0.6 ml. The client should receive _____ ml SC bid.

26. The physician orders ketorolac tromethamine 30 mg IV q6h for 48 hours. The client should receive a total of how many doses of ketorolac tromethamine? _____

27. The physician orders cyanocobalamin 50 mcg IM. The pharmacy sends cyanocobalamin 100 mcg/ml. The client should receive _____ ml IM.

28. The physician orders interferon alfa-2b recombinant 12 million units SC. The pharmacy sends interferon alfa-2b recombinant 10 million units/0.5 ml. The client should receive _____ ml SC.

29. The physician orders cyanocobalamin 0.3 mg IM. The pharmacy sends cyanocobalamin 100 mcg/ 0.5 ml. The client should receive _____ ml IM.

30. The physician orders metoclopramide 25 mg IV bolus as a premed for chemotherapy. The pharmacy supplies metoclopramide 5 mg/ml. The nurse should administer _____ ml slowly IV bolus.

31. The physician orders digoxin 75 mcg IV bolus. The pharmacy supplies digoxin 0.1 mg/ml. The client should receive _____ ml IV bolus.

32. The physician orders digoxin immune Fab 36 mg IV bolus. The pharmacy supplies digoxin immune Fab 10 mg/ml. The client should receive _____ ml IV bolus.

33. The physician orders dexamethasone 8 mg IV bolus. The pharmacy supplies 4 mg/ml dexamethasone. The nurse should administer _____ ml IV bolus as ordered.

34. The physician orders lorazepam 1.5 mg IV bolus. The pharmacy supplies 0.001 g/ml of lorazepam. The nurse should administer _____ ml IV bolus as ordered.

35. The physician orders furosemide 0.04 g IV bolus. The pharmacy sends furosemide 20 mg/ml. The client should receive _____ ml IV bolus.

36. The physician orders acyclovir 350 mg IV. A vial of 500 mg of acyclovir comes in powder form with directions to reconstitute with 5 ml of normal saline. How many milliliters would contain the ordered amount? _____

37. The doctor orders 250 mg of cefazolin IV. A vial containing 500 mg of cefazolin powder has instructions to reconstitute with 2 ml of sterile water. How many milliliters would contain the ordered amount? _____

38. The physician orders 500 mg of ceftazidime IV. The label on the 2 gram vial of ceftazidime reads to reconstitute with 10 ml. How many milliliters would contain the ordered amount? _____

39. The label on the vial 1 g of ampicillin reads to reconstitute with sodium chloride to achieve a concentration of 125 mg/5 ml. How many milliliters of sodium chloride should be added to the vial to achieve this concentration? _____

40. The label on the 1 g powder of azithromycin reads to reconstitute with water to achieve a concentration of 200 mg/5 ml. How many milliliters of water should be added to achieve this concentration? _____

41. The physician orders cefaclor 0.2 g po. The vial of cefaclor powder reads to reconstitute with water to achieve a concentration of 400 mg/ 5 ml. How many milliliters will achieve the ordered dose? _____

42. The label on the vial of ceprozil 250 mg reads to reconstitute with 5 ml of distilled water. This will provide a concentration of _____ mg/ml.

43. The physician orders ceftazidime 1 g IV. The powder for injection of cetazidime is in a vial with instructions to reconstitute with 50 ml of normal saline for injection to achieve a concentration of 10 mg/ml. How many milliliters will be required to achieve the ordered dose? _____

44. The label on the 1 g vial of cephadine powder reads to reconstitute with 40 ml of distilled water for oral suspension. This will provide a concentration of _____ mg/ml.

45. The physician orders clarithromycin 500 mg po bid. The label on the bottle of granules for oral suspension reads to reconstitute with water to achieve a concentration of 0.125 g/5 ml. The nurse should administer _____ ml of reconstituted medication to achieve the ordered dose.

46. The physician orders clindamycin HCl 900 mg IV q8h. The label on the vial of clindamycin powder for injection reads to reconstitute in 5% dextrose to achieve a concentration of 10 gr/50 ml. The nurse will have to infuse _____ ml to administer the ordered dose.

47. A client is to receive coagulation factor VIIA intravenous bolus. It is supplied in powder that is to be reconstituted with sterile water to achieve a concentration of 4.8 mg/8.5 ml. The client weighs 40 kg and his dosage is based on 90 mcg/kg. The nurse should administer _____ ml for the appropriate dose for this client.

48. The physician orders cefoxitin sodium 0.5 g q4h IV. The vial of cefoxitin sodium powder for injection has been reconstituted with sterile water to a concentration of 20 mg/ml. How many milliliters will be needed to achieve the ordered dose? _____

49. The physician orders clindamycin 20 gr IV. The label on the vial of clindamycin powder for injection reads to reconstitute with sterile water to produce a concentration of 600 mg/50 ml. How many milliliters would be required to administer the ordered dose? _____

50. The label on the 25 mg vial of diltiazem HCl powder reads to reconstitute with sterile water to prepare a solution of 5 mg/ml. The nurse must add _____ ml of diluent to this vial to achieve the concentration on the vial.

51. Doctor's order: 1000 ml D_5W to infuse over 8 hours
    Hourly rate: _____

52. Doctor's order: 2000 ml D_5W/½ NS to infuse over 10 hours
    Hourly rate: _____

53. Doctor's order: 250 ml of vancomycin 500 mg to infuse over 90 minutes
    Hourly rate: _____

54. Doctor's order: 50 ml cefazolin sodium 1 gram to infuse over 15 minutes
    Hourly rate: _____

55. Doctor's order: 100 ml gentamycin 80 mg to infuse over 30 minutes
    Hourly rate: _____

56. Doctor's order: 3000 ml of lactated Ringer's to infuse over 12 hours
    Hourly rate: _____

57. Doctor's order: 100 ml ampicillin sodium 500 mg to infuse over 40 minutes
    Hourly rate: _____

58. Doctor's order: 350 ml lactated Ringer's to infuse over 5 hours
    Hourly rate: _____

59. Doctor's order: 320 ml packed red blood cells (blood) to infuse over 4 hours
    Hourly rate: _____

60. Doctor's order: 0.5 L of D_5/½ normal saline with 20 mEq potassium chloride to infuse over 10 hrs
    Hourly rate: _____

61. Doctor's order: 25 ml of ondansetron to infuse over 15 minutes
    Hourly rate: _____

62. Doctor's order: 25 ml of diphenhydramine to infuse over 20 minutes
    Hourly rate: _____

63. Doctor's order: 1000 ml D_5W to infuse over 8 hours
    Drip factor: 20 gtt/ml
    _____ gtt/min

64. Doctor's order: 250 ml NS to infuse over 2 hours
    Drip factor: 10 gtt/ml
    _____ gtt/min

65. Doctor's order: 2000 ml D$_5$W/½ NS to infuse over 10 hours
    Drip factor: 15 gtt/ml
    _____ gtt/min

66. Doctor's order: 1500 ml D$_5$W/¼ NS to infuse over 12 hours
    Drip factor: 10 gtt/ml
    _____ gtt/min

67. Doctor's order: 50 ml cefazolin sodium 1 gram to infuse over 15 minutes
    Drip factor: 10 gtt/ml
    _____ gtt/min

68. Doctor's order: 150 ml of NS to infuse over 4 hours
    Drip factor: 60 gtt/ml
    _____ gtt/min

69. Doctor's order: 65 ml/hr of NS
    Drip factor: 60 gtt/ml
    _____ gtt/min

70. Doctor's order: 50 ml of ceftriaxone sodium 1 g to infuse over 45 minutes
    Hourly rate: _____

71. Doctor's order: 1656 ml of total parenteral nutrition (TPN) to infuse over 24 hours
    Hourly rate: _____

72. Cefdinir is ordered for a child weighing 31 pounds. The safe dosage for cefdinir is 7 mg/kg every 12 hours. What is the safe dose for this child? _____

73. The physician orders azithromycin 200 mg one time dose for a child weighing 44 pounds. The safe dosage is 10 mg/kg of body weight. What is the safe dose for this child? _____ Is this a safe dose for this child? _____

74. The physician orders gentamycin 80 mg IV q8h for a child weighing 22 pounds. The safe dosage range is 6–7.5 mg/kg of body weight/24 hours. What is the safe dosage range/dose for this child? _____ Is the ordered dose safe for this child? _____

75. The safe dosage range for acetaminophen is 10–15 mg/kg of body weight q4h. What is the maximum safe dose for a child weighing 33 pounds? _____

76. The safe dosage range for ibuprofen is 20–40 mg/kg/day. What is the maximum safe dose for a child weighing 25 pounds? _____

77. The safe dosage for cefaclor is 20 mg/kg/day. The physician orders cefaclor 300 mg q8h for a child weighing 40 kg. What is the safe dose for this child? _____ Is the ordered dose safe? _____

78. The physician orders cefazolin sodium 150 mg IV q6h for a child weighing 35 pounds. The safe dosage range for cefazolin sodium is 25–50 mg/kg/day in 4 divided doses. What is the safe individual dose **range** for this child? _____ Is the ordered dose safe? _____

79. Acetaminophen is ordered for a child weighing 14 pounds. The safe dosage range for acetaminophen is 10–15 mg/kg/dose. What is the safe dosage **range** for this child? _____

80. Digoxin is ordered for an infant weighing 9 pounds. The safe dosage range for this drug is 35–60 mcg/kg/dose. What is the safe dosage **range** for this infant? _____

81. Ampicillin sodium IV is ordered for a child weighing 33 pounds. The safe dosage range of this drug is 25–50 mg/kg/24 hours. What is the safe daily dose for this child? _____

82. Aminophylline IV is ordered for a 4-year-old child weighing 31 pounds. The safe dosage range of aminophylline for this age child is 0.8–1.2 mg/kg/hr. What is the safe dosage **range** for this child? _____

83. Clarithromycin is ordered for a child weighing 12 kilograms. The safe dosage of this drug is 15 mg/kg q12h. What is the safe dose of clarithromycin for this child? _____

84. The physician orders diazepam 1 mg po q6h for a child weighing 28 pounds. The safe dose for this drug is 0.5 mg/kg/dose. What is the safe dose for this child? _____ Is the ordered dose safe? _____

85. 1000 ml bag of 5% dextrose in water with 20 meq of potassium chloride is to infuse at 125 ml/hr. How long will this bag last? _____

86. 720 ml of total parenteral nutrition is programmed into the intravenous infusion pump to infuse at 36 ml/hr. How long will this infusion last? _____

87. 25 ml of ondansetron 4 mg is to infuse at 17 gtt/min using a macrodrip tubing with a drip factor of 10 gtt/ml. How long will this infusion last? _____

88. The physician orders oxicillin sodium 500 mg in 50 ml of 5% dextrose/0.9% normal saline to infuse at 100 ml/hr. How long will this infusion last? _____

89. The physician orders vancomycin 750 mg to infuse at 7.5 mg/kg/hr for a client weighing 50 kg. The pharmacy sends 750 mg vancomycin in 250 mg 0.9% normal saline. How long will this infusion last? _____

90. 1000 ml of 5% dextrose in water is to infuse at 50 ml/hr. How long will this infusion last?
_____

91. 180 ml of 20% intralipids is programmed to infuse at 10 ml/hr. How long will this infusion last? _____

92. 1060 ml of total parenteral nutrition is programmed to infuse at 53 ml/hr. How long will this infusion last? _____

93. 600 ml of IV solution is in the IV bag when you start your shift at 0700. The infusion rate is 100 ml/hr. At what time will this infusion be completed? _____

94. When you begin your shift at 0700, the client's enteral feeding bag contains 240 ml. The physician's order reads to start enteral feedings at 30 ml/hr and q2h increase the feeding by 10 ml until a goal of 80 ml/hr. At what time will this feeding be completed?
_____

95. The physician orders regular insulin to infuse intravenously at 10 units/hour. The pharmacy sends 100 units of regular insulin in 500 ml of 0.9% normal saline. The intravenous infusion pump should be programmed to infuse how many milliliters/hour to deliver the ordered dose? _____

96. The physician orders heparin sodium to infuse intravenously at 1100 units/hr. The pharmacy sends 25,000 units of heparin in 500 ml of ½ normal saline solution. The intravenous infusion pump should be programmed to infuse how many milliliters/hour to deliver the ordered dose? _____

97. The physician orders heparin sodium to infuse intravenously at 800 units/hr. The pharmacy sends 20,000 units of heparin in 500 ml of 0.9% normal saline solution. The intravenous infusion pump should be programmed to infuse how many ml/hour to deliver the ordered dose? _____

98. The physician orders potassium chloride to infuse at 10 mEq/hour. The pharmacy sends 50 mEq of potassium chloride in 250 ml of 5% dextrose in water. The intravenous infusion pump should be programmed to infuse how many ml/hr to deliver the ordered dose? _____

99. Aminophylline 500 mg in 1000 ml of 5% dextrose in water to infuse at 25 mg/hr. The intravenous infusion pump should be programmed to infuse how many ml/hr to deliver the ordered dose? _____

100. The physician orders regular insulin 5 units per hour intravenous to be administered at a rate of 25 ml/hr. Available is 500 ml of 0.9% normal saline and a vial of regular insulin. How many units of insulin would you add to the IV solution to deliver the ordered rate?

_____

101. The physician orders morphine sulfate 4 mg/hr intravenously. The pharmacy sends morphine sulfate 50 mg in 500 ml of 5% dextrose in water. How many ml/hr should be infused to deliver to ordered rate? _____

Answers for Unit X

1. 2 capsules
2. 3 tablets
3. 1 capsule
4. 1 tablet
5. 1 tablet
6. 2 tablets
7. 1 tablet
8. 1 tablet
9. 12 tablets
10. 2 ml
11. 4.5 ml
12. 3 ml
13. 5 ml
14. 13.3 ml
15. 2.5 ml
16. 20 ml
17. 7.5 ml
18. 10 ml
19. 1.5 ml
20. 44 units
21. 1 ml
22. 35 ml
23. 0.25 ml
24. 11 ml
25. 0.3 ml
26. 8 doses
27. 0.5 ml
28. 0.6 ml
29. 1.5 ml
30. 5 ml
31. 0.75 ml
32. 3.6 ml
33. 2.0 ml
34. 1.5 ml
35. 2.0 ml
36. 3.5 ml
37. 1.0 ml
38. 2.5 ml
39. 40 ml
40. 25 ml
41. 2.5 ml
42. 50 mg/ml
43. 100 ml
44. 25 mg/ml
45. 20 ml
46. 75 ml
47. 6.4 ml
48. 25 ml
49. 100 ml
50. 5 ml
51. 125 ml/hr
52. 200 ml/hr
53. 167 ml/hr
54. 200 ml/hr

55. 200 ml/hr
56. 250 ml/hr
57. 150 ml/hr
58. 70 ml/hr
59. 80 ml/hr
60. 50 ml/hr
61. 100 ml/hr
62. 75 ml/hr
63. 42 gtt/min
64. 21 gtt/min
65. 50 gtt/min
66. 21 gtt/min
67. 33 gtt/min
68. 38 gtt/min
69. 65 gtt/min
70. 66.7 ml/hr
71. 69 ml/hr
72. 98.6 mg/dose
73. 200 mg/dose; Yes, dose safe.
74. 20–25 mg/dose; No, dose not safe.
75. 225 mg/dose
76. 454.5 mg/day
77. 266.7 mg/dose; No, dose not safe.
78. 99.4–198.9 mg/dose; Yes, dose safe.
79. 63.6–95.5 mg/dose
80. 143.2–244.5 mcg/dose
81. 375–750 mg/day
82. 11.3–16.9 mg/hr
83. 180 mg q12h
84. 6.4 mg/dose q12h; Yes, dose safe.
85. 8 hrs.
86. 20 hrs.
87. 15 min
88. 30 min
89. 2 hr
90. 20 hr
91. 18 hr
92. 20 hr
93. 1300 or 1:00 pm
94. 1300 or 1:00 pm
95. 50 ml/hr
96. 22 ml/hr
97. 20 ml/hr
98. 50 ml/hr
99. 50 ml/hr
100. 100 units
101. 40 ml/hr

References

Food and Drug Administration (FDA). http://www.fda.gov

Gahart, B. L. and Nazareno, A. R. (2002). *2002 Intravenous medications*. (18th ed). St. Louis, MO: Mosby/Harcourt Health Sciences.

Mayo Clinic Medical Center. http://www.mayoclinic.org

Nurse's PDR Resource Center. http://www.NursesPDR.com

Olsen, J. L. and Giangrasso, A. P. (2000). *Medical dosage calculations*. (7th ed.). Upper Saddle River, NJ: Prentice Hall Health.

Pickar, G. D. (1999). *Dosage calculations*. (6th ed.). Clifton Park, NY: Delmar Learning.

Reiss, B. S., Evans, M. E., and Broyles, B. E. (2002). *Pharmacological aspects of nursing care.* (6th ed.). Clifton Park, NY: Delmar Learning.

Saxton, D. F. and O'Neill, N. E. (1998). *Math and Meds for Nurses.* Clifton Park, NY: Delmar Learning.

Spratto, G. R. and Woods, A. L. (2002). *PDR: Nurse's drug handbook.* Clifton Park, NY: Delmar Learning.

U.S. Pharmaceuticals. http://www.usp.org/